W9-ABS-027

HIGH INTENSITY INTERVAL TRAINING FOR WOMEN

Publisher: Mike Sanders
Executive Managing Editor: Billy Fields
Senior Acquisitions Editor: Brook Farling
Development Editor: Ann Barton
Senior Production Editor: Janette Lynn
Cover Designer: Nicola Powling
Book Designer: XAB Design
Photographer: Matt Bowen
Indexer: Johnna Vanhoose Dinse
Layout: Ayanna Lacey
Proofreader: Laura Caddell

First American Edition, 2015

DK Publishing
345 Hudson Street
New York, New York 10014

15   16   17   18   19   10   9   8   7   6   5   4   3   2   1

01–282775–Jan/2015

Copyright © 2015 Dorling Kindersley Limited
All rights reserved.

Without limiting the rights under copyright reserved above, no part of this publication
may be reproduced, stored in or introduced into a retrieval system, or transmitted, in
any form, or by any means (electronic, mechanical, photocopying, recording, or
otherwise), without the prior written permission of both the copyright owner and the
above publisher of this book.

Published in Great Britain by Dorling Kindersley Limited.

A catalog record for this book is available from the Library of Congress.

ISBN 978-1-4654-3535-4

Note: The techniques, ideas and suggestions presented in this book are intended to
provide helpful and information are not meant to substitute for the advice of a health
care professional. It is recommended that the reader consult with their physician or
health care professional before beginning this or any other new exercise program. The
author and publisher assume no responsibility for any injuries suffered following the
training outlined in this book and specifically disclaim any responsibility for any
liability, loss, or risk, personal or otherwise, which is incurred as a consequence,
directly or indirectly, of the use and application of any of the contents of this book.

DK books are available at special discounts when purchased in bulk for sales
promotions, premiums, fund-raising, or educational use. For details, contact:
DK Publishing Special Markets, 345 Hudson Street, New York, NY 10014 or
SpecialSales@dk.com.

Printed and bound in the United States by Courier Kendallville

www.dk.com

A WORLD OF IDEAS:
SEE ALL THERE IS TO KNOW

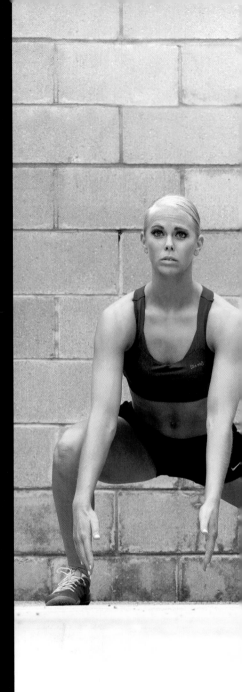

HIGH INTENSITY INTERVAL TRAINING FOR WOMEN

BURN MORE FAT in LESS TIME with HIIT WORKOUTS YOU CAN DO ANYWHERE

 Sean Bartram

Official Trainer to the Indianapolis Colts Cheerleaders

WITHDRAWN FROM
RAPIDES PARISH LIBRARY
RAPIDES PARISH LIBRARY

CONTENTS

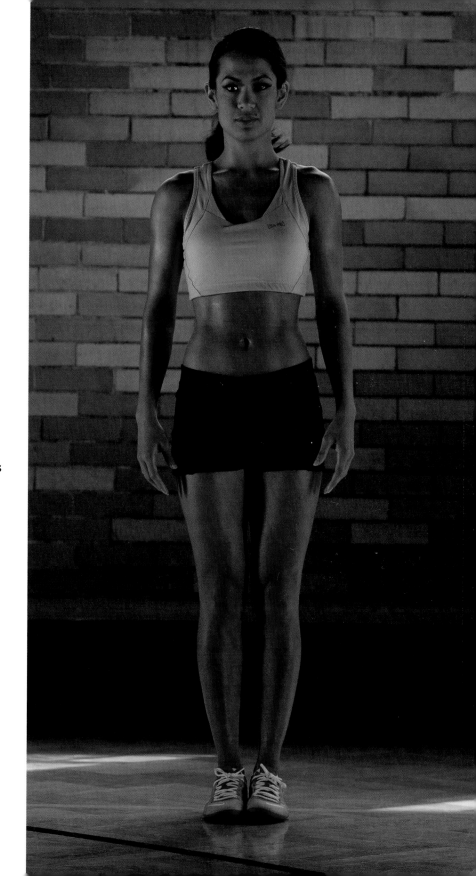

INTRODUCTION

High-intensity interval training (HIIT) is on fire right now. Why is it so popular? We live in a society where every second needs to count or be accounted for. We lead busy lives and we want more bang for our buck, but in half the time. Unlike many things in life, HIIT can deliver on its promises.

If you can give me everything you've got for 20 minutes, I will give you a workout that will fire up your metabolism for 48 hours, help you defy age, build strength, increase definition, and improve your heart health.

As a master trainer for celebrity fitness instructor Tracy Anderson and now as official trainer to the Indianapolis Colts Cheerleaders and owner of Core Pilates and Fitness, I am tasked with helping people from all walks of life get fit, lose weight, and improve their overall health and fitness. No matter the end goal, I have successfully used the exercises and routines in this book to help my clients reach their peak physical fitness. If you put forth the effort, I know this book and HIIT can empower you to meet your fitness goals, too.

With 60 exercises and over 50 unique routines that range from four minutes to an hour in length, this book provides all the information and resources you need to make HIIT part of your fitness routine, regardless of your goals or starting point.

Turn the page to learn more about HIIT and enter the exciting world of "Leg Hell" and "Metabolic Mayhem." This book will challenge you mentally and physically, but remember: good things come to those who SWEAT!

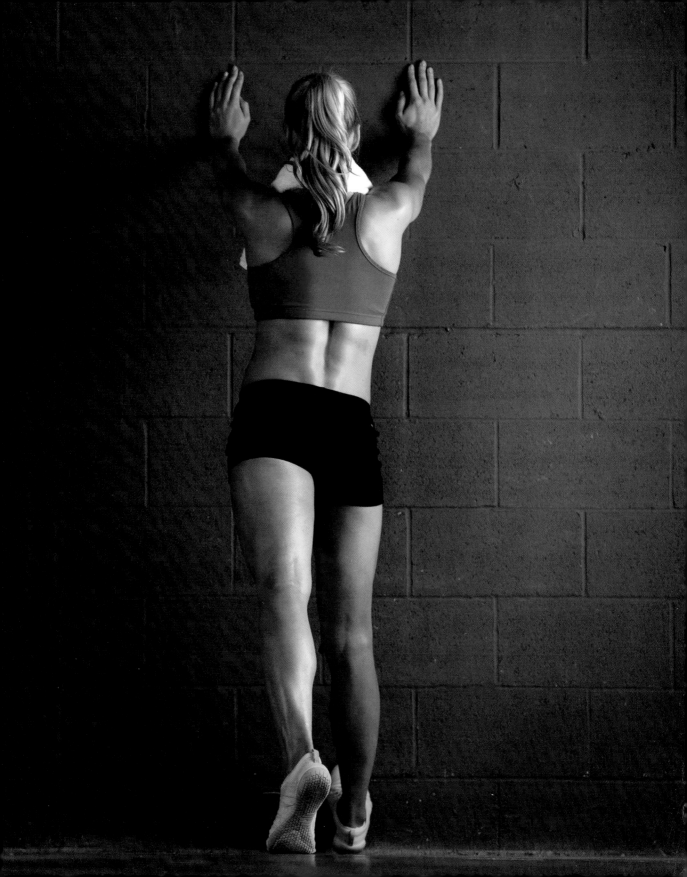

USING THIS BOOK

As with any exercise program, HIIT is not without risk. I strongly recommend that you consult a physician or primary health-care provider before undertaking this or any exercise program.

The use of this book is determined by your end goal. If weight loss, fat burning, increased muscle tone, and definition are your goal, the routines and programs in this book will help you meet it. If you're looking to supplement your existing workout regimen, increase your athletic performance, or are simply intrigued by HIIT, you'll find inspiration and learn some new exercises to add to your arsenal.

FITNESS ASSESSMENT

In order to get to where you want to be, you have to know where you're starting. The fitness assessment in this book is not intended to recommend a particular course of action regarding your health, but it is meant to give you a sense of your current fitness level and provide a basis for you to create your fitness goals.

The assessment is comprised of four foundational exercises. Your performance on these exercises will allow you to quickly and easily determine the level at which you should be working out. Once you've committed to a workout regimen, reassess your fitness every couple of weeks to track your progress and up the intensity if necessary.

ROUTINES

At the core of this book are 50 routines that range in length from four minutes to one hour, beginning with easier routines and progressing to those that are more challenging. Most routines supply three levels of difficulty, designated either by work-to-rest ratio, difficulty of the exercises, or number of repetitions.

Level 1: If you're new to HIIT or just getting back into working out after a long hiatus, this level is for you.

Level 2: This is the intermediate level. It's best for those who work out relatively regularly but aren't quite ready for the intensity of Level 3.

Level 3: This level is for those who are in shape and looking for a challenge.

PROGRAMS

For those looking for a more structured approach, consider committing to one of the HIIT programs. These programs range from 3 to 28 days in length and will give you a set schedule for completing your HIIT routines.

EXERCISES

To keep HIIT interesting, you need a variety of effective and challenging exercises. This book includes step-by-step instructions for each of the 60 exercises used in the routines. If you're not familiar with an exercise, check the instructions and practice it a few times to master the form before using it regularly.

The exercises are grouped by primary focus (cardio, core, lower body, and upper body), but many challenge multiple muscle groups and provide cardiovascular benefits. If you're feeling adventurous, try creating your own routines by combining several exercises.

COMMITMENT AND EFFORT

As with most things, the saying "you get out what you put in" is absolutely true for HIIT. Your body will only go where your mind pushes it. If you only give 50 percent of the effort required, you can only expect 50 percent of the result. The key to HIIT is truly pushing yourself to the limit during the high-intensity intervals.

You might think pushing yourself means going through the workout as quickly as possible. It's true that speed is important, but form trumps speed. Focus on quality, not quantity, to get the most out of the exercises and routines.

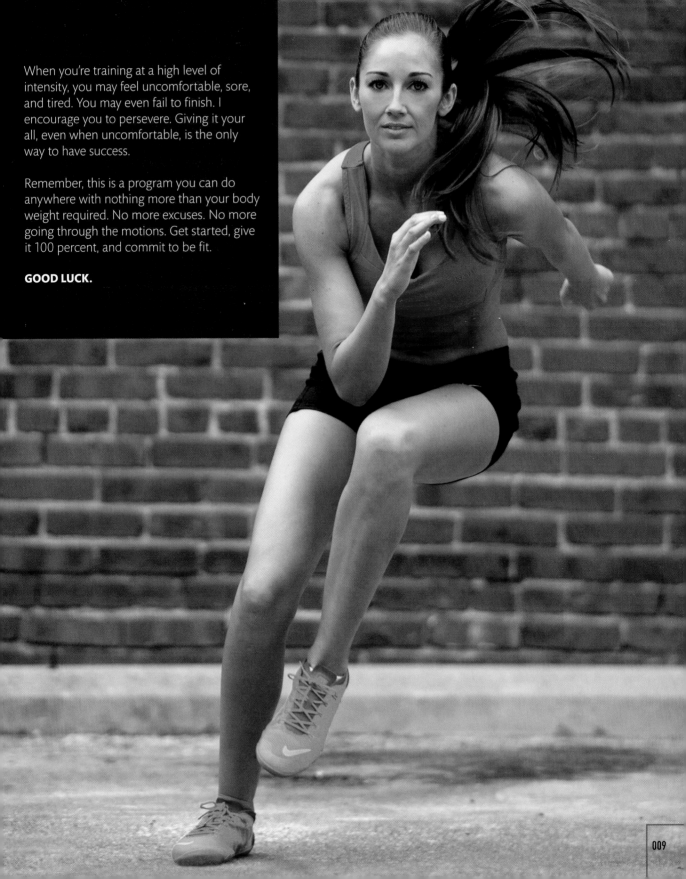

When you're training at a high level of intensity, you may feel uncomfortable, sore, and tired. You may even fail to finish. I encourage you to persevere. Giving it your all, even when uncomfortable, is the only way to have success.

Remember, this is a program you can do anywhere with nothing more than your body weight required. No more excuses. No more going through the motions. Get started, give it 100 percent, and commit to be fit.

GOOD LUCK.

MEET THE MODELS

The four models featured in the book are current squad members of the Indianapolis Colts Cheerleaders. In that role, they have entertained troops across the globe, raised thousands of dollars for cancer research, and represented the Indianapolis Colts across four continents.

As cheerleaders, they must maintain peak physical fitness to power through their rigorous routines. HIIT gives them a workout that keeps them athletic, fit, and looking amazing. Their toned muscles are the result of hard work, consistent effort, and HIIT workouts.

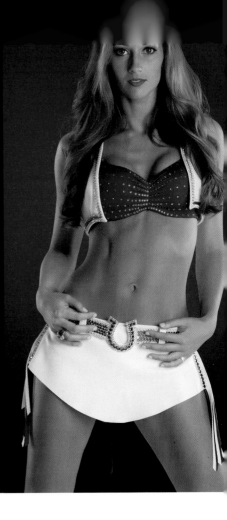

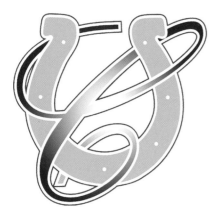

BREANNA

has been with the Colts for six seasons. During that time, she has traveled to Mexico, Japan, and China. She's also cheered at Super Bowl XLIV and was selected as a ProBowl cheerleader in 2013. A graduate of Ball State University, she now has a career in human resources. She loves HIIT because it's a fantastic cardio workout and delivers results. Her HIIT advice: "Love your body! Hydrate it, nourish it, and maintain it, but above all else LOVE you!"

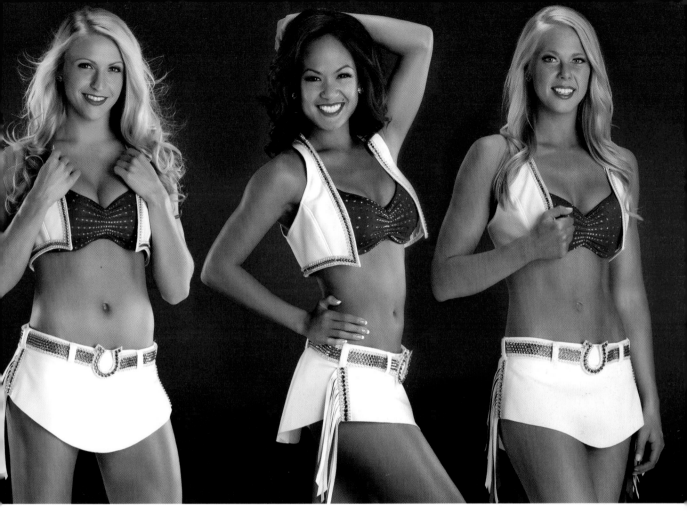

BRITTANY

has been a Colts cheerleader for three years and she still gets a rush each time she runs onto the field to cheer on the team. Her favorite thing about HIIT is the variety; every single time you can expect something different and fun. Her HIIT advice: "Don't give up. When you first start doing HIIT, there may be sometimes where you need a break—it's okay! Do it every day if you can, and don't get discouraged if it is more difficult than you expected when you are first getting started. The more you do it, the easier it gets and the more fun it gets."

CRYSTAL ANNE

has been cheering for the Colts for four years. During that time, she has danced in a Super Bowl music video, volunteered for many charities, undertaken a military tour to entertain troops and their families, and even shaved her head to help raise funds for cancer research in 2013. Her passion for health and fitness has led to a career as a personal trainer at the National Institute for Fitness and Sport (NIFS). Her HIIT advice: "Quality over quantity! Perform the exercise correctly with full function and form before adding in your speed, and have fun!"

ERIN

has been on the squad for five years. Some of her cheerleading highlights include appearing on the Jimmy Fallon show and traveling to London for NFL UK. Erin is also a trainer at Core Fitness and Pilates, where she teaches HIIT as well as Pilates reformer classes and TRX. Practicing HIIT makes her feel fit, confident, and athletic. Her HIIT advice: "Keep moving! It's not easy at first, but if you keep moving and try your hardest, you will become better and better. Always push yourself; that's the only way to keep improving!"

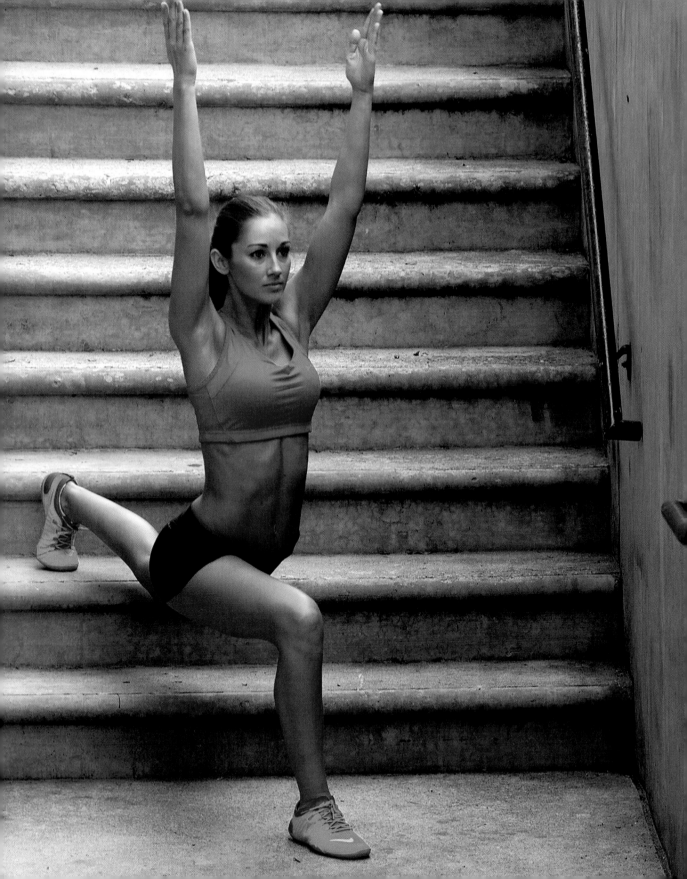

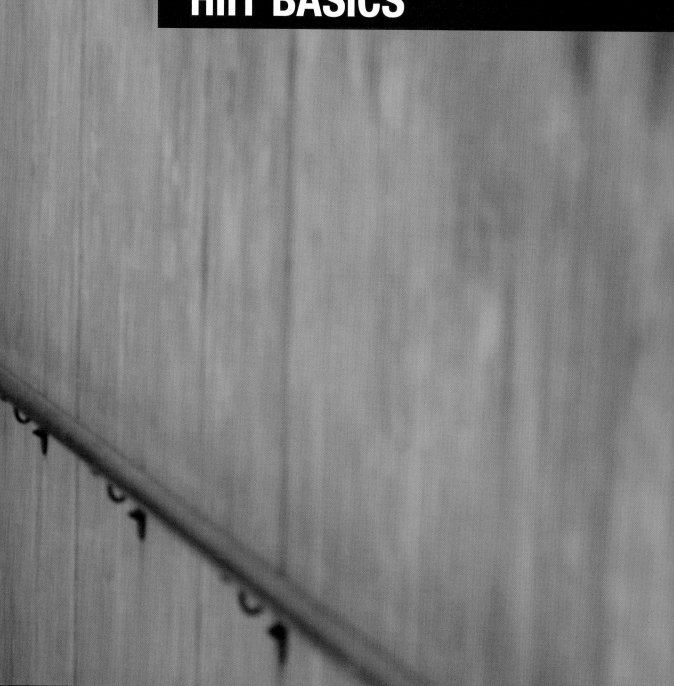

HIIT BASICS

01

WHAT IS HIIT?

High-intensity interval training, or HIIT, has exploded in recent years due to its promise of an efficient and effective way to meet fitness goals. Different trainers and instructors approach HIIT in different ways, but at its core, HIIT should always involve alternating short intervals of high-intensity, all-out exercise with short intervals of rest or active recovery. The HIIT principles can be applied to many types of exercise, provided you're able to really elevate your heart rate during the cardio intervals. You could alternate 30 seconds of sprinting with 30 seconds of walking, or you could engage in a series of bodyweight exercises, such as push-ups, doing each for 30 seconds with 10 seconds of rest in between.

What many people love about HIIT is that it's fast. If you're willing to truly push yourself, you can squeeze an effective workout into 10 minutes.

HIIT VS. TRADITIONAL CARDIO WORKOUTS

People spend hours and hours each week engaged in low-intensity cardio activities such as riding a stationary bike, jogging on a treadmill, or using an elliptical machine. Although they're actively burning calories, many people find they're unable to lose significant weight. This is because the body eventually reaches a "steady state." It adjusts to the workload and tries hard to conserve energy (calories).

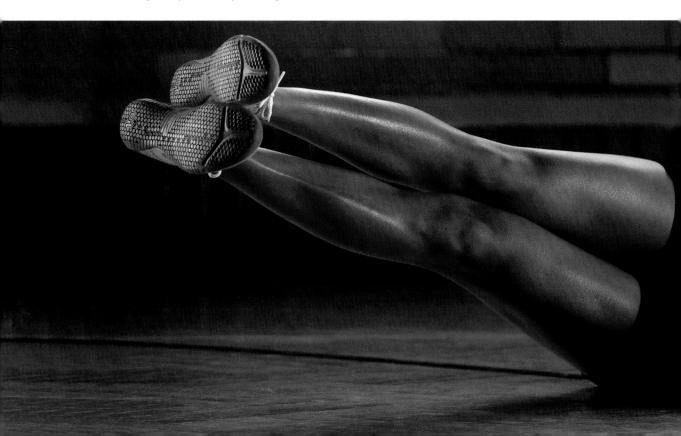

Studies suggest that HIIT is much more effective than traditional cardio activities for burning fat and increasing both aerobic and anaerobic endurance. Alternating between bursts of high output cardio and resistance-based strength exercises means you are constantly keeping your body in a state of confusion, preventing it from adapting to the workload. HIIT also offers you the "after burn" effect, burning calories long after your workout is complete, unlike steady state training.

HIIT FOR WOMEN

The HIIT exercises and routines in this book reflect the approach my staff and I have developed and refined specifically to get the Colts cheerleaders into swimsuit-calendar shape. The exercises target the muscles many women would like to see toned and defined, including the arms, stomach, and legs.

In addition to burning fat and creating definition, I am committed to making my clients stronger, balanced, athletic, and agile. To do this I blend bodyweight resistance, plyometrics (jumping exercises), and unilateral exercises into the routines.

My goal is to stimulate as many muscles as possible during each routine without overloading a particular muscle group. I like to change the elevation of the exercises frequently to drive up the heart rate (for example, transitioning from push-ups to squat jumps). As you stand up, the heart has to work against gravity to get the blood pumped through the body and back to the heart. It beats faster to overcome the effects of gravity.

I also like to mix in multiplanar exercises to improve balance and athletic performance. Multiplanar exercises are any exercise where different joints of the body move through multiple planes of motion at the same time.

COMMIT TO HIIT

The most important aspect of HIIT is committing to the challenge. HIIT is hard. It takes a great deal of determination to sustain the level of output required to succeed. You will be sore, you will want to quit, and you may even fail at times. When this happens, remind yourself why you started HIIT in the first place. Focus on your goals and power through. If you work hard, you will see results.

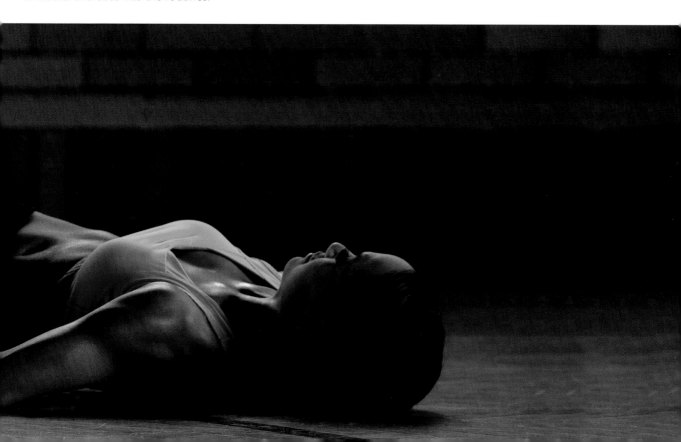

HOW HIIT WORKS

Although short in duration, HIIT has a big impact. Training at your maximum capacity for intense intervals interspersed with rest or active recovery will accomplish two goals: it will help accelerate fat loss and improve both aerobic and anaerobic endurance. HIIT causes your body to burn calories and lose fat in less time than traditional "steady state" training.

HIGH INTENSITY

The "high intensity" part of HIIT is key. You won't see results if you're not pushing yourself as hard as you possibly can during the "work" intervals of your HIIT routine. Studies have shown that just seven minutes of HIIT can create changes in your muscles at a molecular level that are comparable to what you might see after an hour or more of jogging or biking. However, those changes are not apparent if you don't work at maximum output.

CONSTANT CHANGE

The "interval" part of HIIT is also critical. This comes into play with both the brief rest periods between exercises as well as the order of exercises themselves. As you go through a HIIT routine, you alternate between periods of all-out exertion and active recovery or rest. The brief rest periods allow your heart rate to come down and prevent your body from adapting to a steady workload.

THE "AFTER BURN" EFFECT

Not only will you burn calories and fat during your HIIT workout, you will also burn calories and fat following your workout through the "after burn" effect or EPOC (excess post-exercise oxygen consumption). EPOC is the measurable increased rate of oxygen intake following strenuous activity intended to erase the body's oxygen debt.

In order to erase the oxygen debt, fatty acids are released and used as fuel for recovery. You cannot take advantage of this after burn by doing low-intensity exercise. Only by working anaerobically at maximal heart rate will you see this added fat loss effect. EPOC has been shown to last over 48 hours.

ARE YOU WORKING HARD ENOUGH?

Because maximum effort is so critical to HIIT success, my clients often ask, "How do I know if I am working hard enough?" My usual answer is that if the person next to you asks you a question, you should not be able to respond. You should be able to talk between short gasps of air, but if you can carry on a conversation, you're simply not working hard enough.

Another way to think of it is by measuring your workout intensity on a scale of 1 to 10, with 10 equal to running for your life as you are chased by a rabid beast. You should be working almost that hard during a HIIT workout, pushing yourself to a level 8 or 9. Remember that HIIT is hard. Your heart should be pounding, your breathing should be heavy, and you should be sweating.

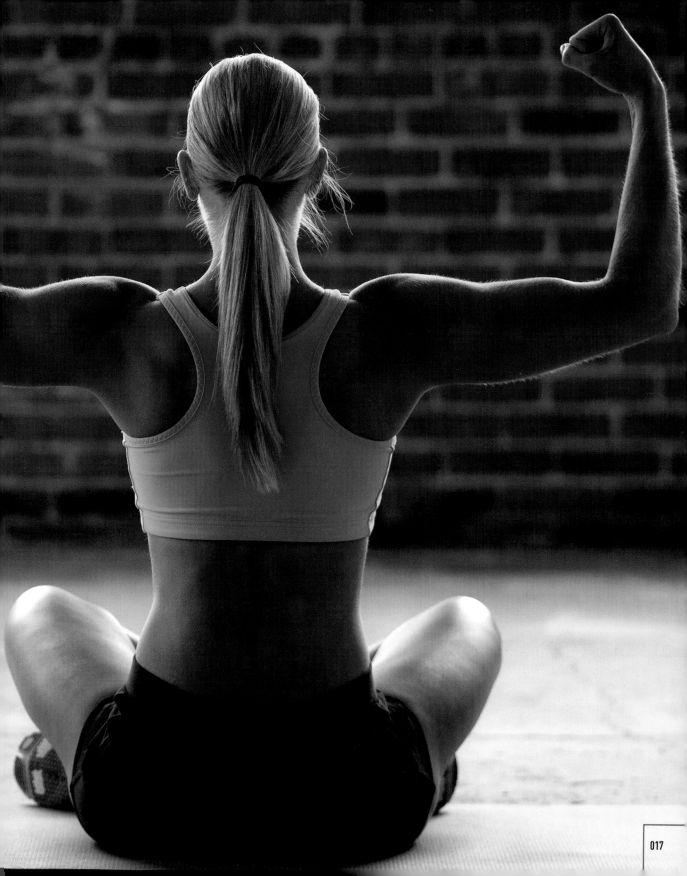

HIIT BENEFITS

HIIT may seem too good to be true. The idea that you can work out for a shorter period of time and see greater health gains than you would with a traditional workout is counterintuitive. However, scientific studies back up the results I see in the studio.

EFFECTIVE WEIGHT LOSS

One reason HIIT is so popular is that it promises measurable and sustainable weight loss. If you're willing to work hard and monitor your nutrition, HIIT really is more effective than other forms of exercise for losing weight. One 1994 study at Laval University in Quebec, Canada, found that HIIT was nine times more effective for losing fat than steady state cardio, such as jogging. This is because HIIT burns fat not only while you're working out, but also for up to 48 hours after exercising through EPOC, also called the "after burn" effect.

FAST, FLEXIBLE, AND FUN

Most HIIT workouts last 30 minutes or less and can be done anywhere, making HIIT the perfect choice for those who don't have the time or opportunity to squeeze in a full hour at the gym every day. With HIIT you have dozens of exercises to choose from that can be combined in countless ways. The ever-changing format of these HIIT routines will provide a unique and fun stimulus.

HIIT is also flexible; it can be done anywhere and requires no equipment. The exercises in this book rely on body weight resistance with an emphasis on achieving maximal heart rate.

LOSE FAT, NOT MUSCLE

If you've ever dieted, you know it's hard not to lose muscle mass along with fat. Studies show that HIIT workouts allow the preservation of muscle mass while losing weight through fat loss. This is because HIIT boosts testosterone and human growth hormone (HGH) levels, which are responsible for lean muscle gain and fat loss. HIIT stimulates the production of HGH by up to 450 percent during the 24 hours after you finish your workout. HGH is not only responsible for increasing your metabolism and stoking your fat burning furnace, but also slows down the aging process.

IMPROVED HEART HEALTH

Most people have never worked as hard as a HIIT demands. Pushing yourself into an anaerobic zone, where it feels like your heart is beating out of your chest, can actually improve your aerobic and anaerobic endurance. A 2012 study published in the *Journal of Strength and Conditioning Research* found that just six HIIT workouts performed over two or three weeks, each lasting only a few minutes, produced measurable improvements in key markers of cardiovascular health.

MITOCHONDRIAL GROWTH

The mitochondria are the power plants of your cells. These tiny cellular structures supply the cell's energy and are also involved with regulating cell growth. How does this relate to HIIT? In 2012, the *American Journal of Physiology* published an article stating that HIIT triggers mitochondrial biogenesis, the process by which new mitochondria are formed within a cell. Mitochondrial biogenesis begins to decline with age, so the ability of HIIT to trigger this process could be described as age-defying.

This was not the first time research has linked exercise to mitochondrial changes. A 2011 study found that exercise induces changes in mitochondrial enzyme content and activity, which can increase your cellular energy production and in so doing decrease your risk of chronic disease. Mitochondrial changes may also benefit your liver, brain, and kidneys.

BENEFITS BEYOND HIIT

HIIT is an incredibly challenging workout when performed to the best of your ability. There are times when you will be uncomfortable, sore, and find it very hard to continue. This is also why HIIT is so rewarding; it not only challenges you physically, but also mentally. Learning to push through the barriers and "suck it up" will enable you to strive for success in all areas of your life, not just your fitness.

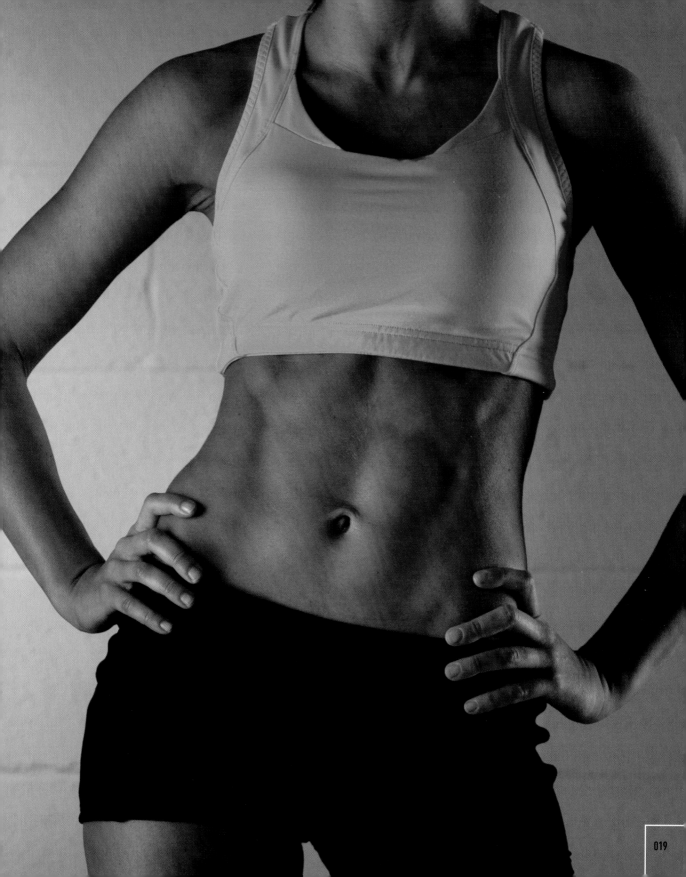

NUTRITION FOR HIIT

Successful high-intensity interval training requires proper nutrition to ensure your body has enough fuel to power you through the HIIT workout.

BEFORE YOUR WORKOUT

As you go through a routine, your body uses stored glycogen along with carbohydrates ingested before the workout for fuel. A typical pre-HIIT meal should be light and provide a good balance of carbs and protein that will help fuel your workout. Don't eat anything too heavy or large; make this pre-workout snack approximately 200 to 300 calories. Good options include:

- Cereal with low-fat milk
- Bagel thin with nut butter spread
- Smoothie with low-fat dairy and fruit

AFTER YOUR WORKOUT

Post workout, it is important to replenish your body with protein and carbohydrates to aid in the repair and recovery process. Within 30 minutes of completing a HIIT workout, try to eat a meal that includes complex carbohydrates and a high protein content such as $\frac{1}{3}$ cup cooked brown rice or quinoa, 1 cup cooked vegetables (2 cups raw), and 3 to 5 ounces of cooked chicken breast. The carbohydrates will replenish your glycogen stores, the main source of fuel for your muscles, and the antioxidants and protein in the chicken will aid in the repair of muscle damage.

DURING THE DAY

You'll get the most out of your HIIT workouts if you eat simple, balanced meals in reasonable portions. I suggest eating lean meat, seafood, vegetables, fruits, whole grains, beans, low-fat dairy foods, and healthy mono-unsaturated fats such as nuts, avocados, and olive oil. I also recommend avoiding sugar and processed foods. This is an eating plan that works for everyone, just adjust the serving sizes according to your needs.

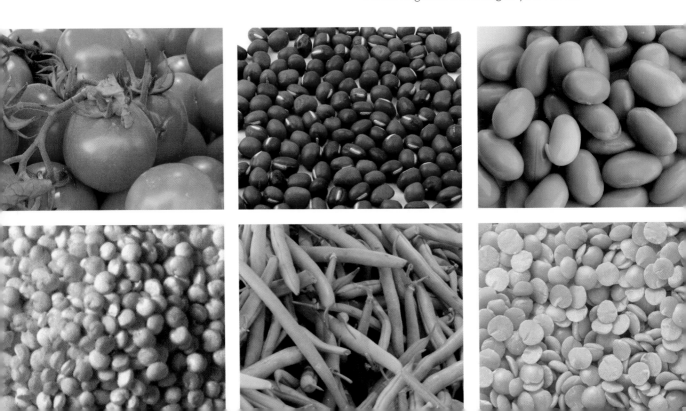

FOR WEIGHT LOSS

If weight loss is your goal, then you need to be aware of your caloric intake. HIIT provides a great fat-burning workout, but at the end of the day, weight loss comes down to a very simple equation: calories in versus calories out. The quality of those calories is also important. While diet choices are a personal decision, I advocate following a few simple guidelines if you're trying to lose weight.

1 Eat three meals a day.
2 Eat two to three smaller snacks between meals, such as protein shakes, raw vegetables, or almonds. These snacks should be 100 to 200 calories.
3 Make sure your meals and snacks contain a good source and supply of lean protein—it's the building block of muscle.
4 Avoid foods made with white sugar and flour. Following this guideline will help you stay away from highly processed, simple carbohydrates that the body quickly turns to fat.
5 Cut out alcohol.
6 Limit your carbohydrates to unprocessed, complex carbs, such as sweet potatoes.
7 Eliminate soda, sweetened coffee beverages, and other high-calorie, sugary drinks.
8 Drink lots of water. It will help flush toxins from your body and keep you feeling satiated.

HYDRATING

Proper hydration is vital to your athletic performance and health. To perform your best, you need to take in an adequate amount of fluid before, during, and after your workouts. Just a 2 percent decrease in bodyweight caused by dehydration can reduce athletic performance by 20 percent.

Thirty minutes before your workout, consume 5 to 10 ounces of a sports drink that is high in electrolytes including sodium, potassium, magnesium, and chloride. Your hydration needs during your workout will depend on the duration and intensity of your activities. One common suggestion is to weigh yourself before a long, intense workout and drink 16 ounces of fluid for every pound lost during the workout.

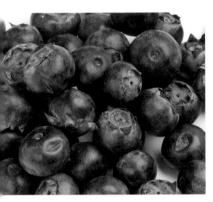
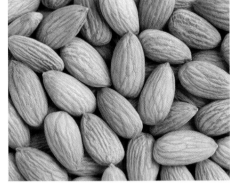
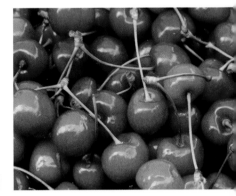
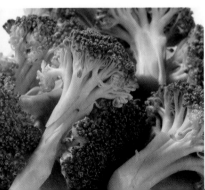
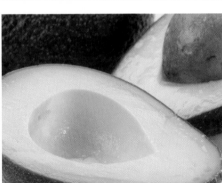
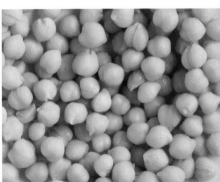

WHAT YOU'LL NEED

The beauty of HIIT is that you need little more than your body and a great attitude to get an incredible workout. However, there are a few things I suggest for optimal performance and comfort during the routines.

FOOTWEAR

During your workout, it's important to consider the placement of your feet on the floor. You need to keep the pad of your big toe, the pad of your little toe, and your heel on the floor. If the pad of your big toe lifts, you have a tendency to roll your weight to the outside (oversupination). If the pad of your little toe lifts, you roll inward (overpronation). Both of these positions will lead to an unstable base of support and could cause injury.

To make you more aware of your foot position, I advocate using a minimalist shoe when training. Two styles I recommend are the Nike Free 1.0 Cross Bionic, specifically designed for HIIT with a lower profile, and INOV-8's F-Lite range of shoes. If you're new to minimalist footwear, it's best to alternate between your old shoes and the minimalist shoes for about two weeks, allowing your body to adjust to the decrease in cushioning and support.

YOGA MAT

You may wish to use a yoga mat for floor exercises. This will provide traction and may be more comfortable for exercises done on the back. I use The Mat by Lululemon (lululemon.com) in the studio with my clients, because I like its reversible surface.

WATCH OR TIMER

A watch or timer is essential for keeping track of the work and rest intervals during HIIT routines. Use whatever is comfortable and easy to operate, whether it's a sport watch, heart rate monitor, or a smartphone app. The app I prefer to use in studio is the Interval Timer Pro, which allows you to program routines and save them for future use.

TOWEL

It's always good to keep a towel on hand during HIIT routines. I expect you to be sweaty, and you will want to dry not only your hands and brow but also the surface on which you are performing the routines to avoid slip and fall injuries.

FOAM ROLLER

An inexpensive tool that you will learn to love, foam rollers provide myofascial release in much the same way as static stretching and massage. Use of a foam roller can prevent injury and speed recovery post-workout.

OPTIONAL EXTRAS

HIIT is about using as many muscle groups as possible in unison during fast explosive exercises. Adding weights or performing isolation exercises, such as bicep curls, can be prohibitive. However, for some core exercises, it's okay to challenge yourself by incorporating added weight. You can add resistance to exercises like Russian twists, V-ups, and sprinter sit-ups with a dumbbell, kettlebell, or medicine ball.

I also highly recommend a product called SandBells from Hyperwear (hyperwear.com). These weights contain sand, which shifts with your movements, challenging your balance and making your workout more effective. Hyperwear also makes a product called Hyper-Vest Pro. This weighted vest adds 10 pounds of evenly distributed weight to the torso and is a safe and effective way to add resistance to every exercise in this book.

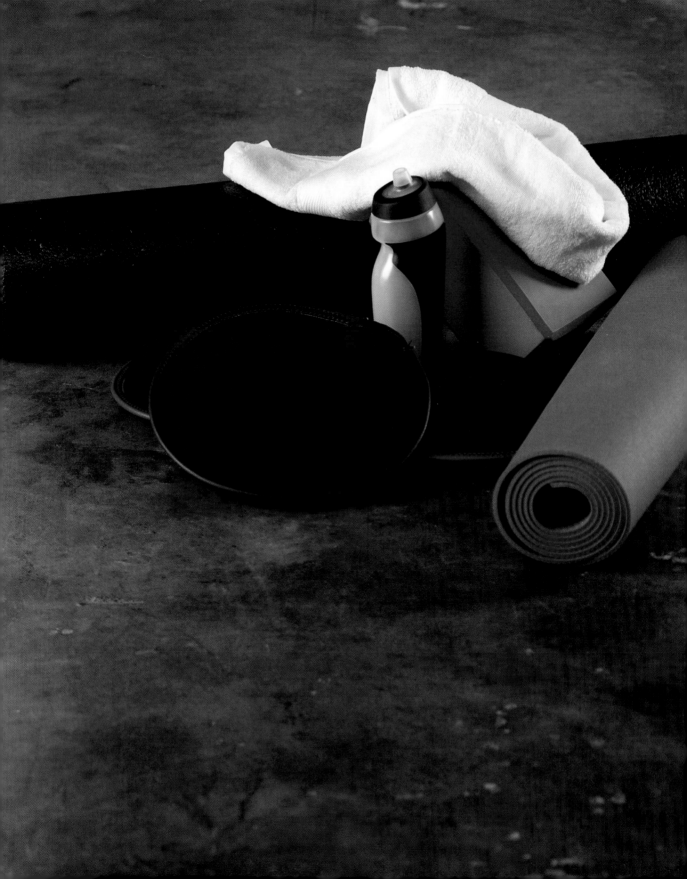

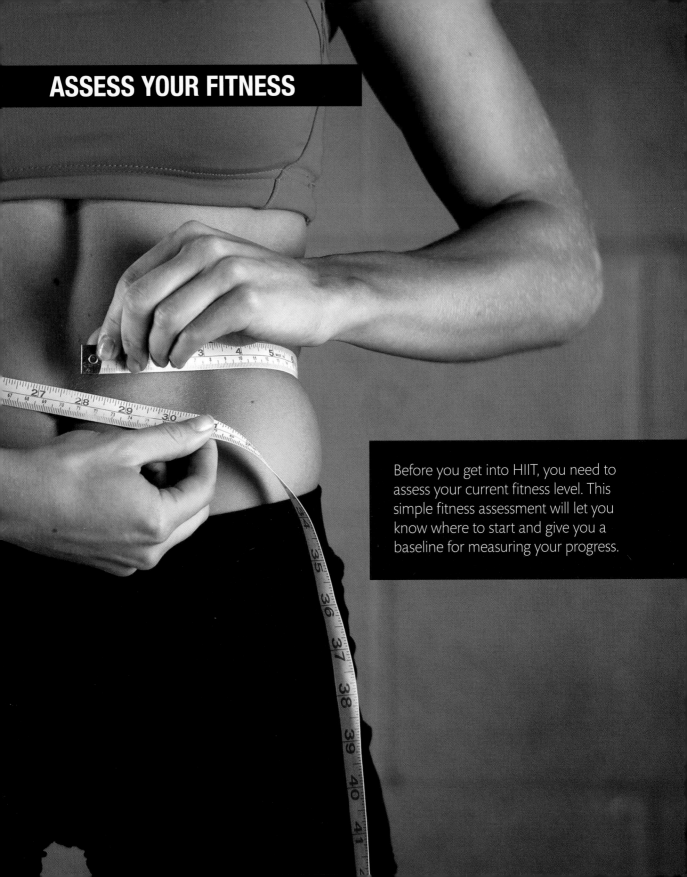

ASSESS YOUR FITNESS

Before you get into HIIT, you need to assess your current fitness level. This simple fitness assessment will let you know where to start and give you a baseline for measuring your progress.

The fitness assessment consists of four basic exercises: **x-jacks**, **push-ups**, **squats**, and **sprinter sit-ups**. Before you begin, review the instructions for each exercise, then follow these steps:

1 Do each exercise for 30 seconds.
2 Rest for 30 seconds after each exercise.
3 Record the number of reps you were able to do of each exercise during the 30-second interval (for example, 20 squats).
4 Add up the total number of reps completed for all exercises to get your total score.

If your score is ...
0-80 Begin with the Level 1 routines.
81-104 Begin with the Level 2 routines.
105 or higher Begin with the Level 3 routines.

Use this assessment as a tool to track your progress and to know when you're ready to tackle the next level by reassessing every 14 days.

BODY FAT PERCENTAGE

A body fat test is an attempt to separate every pound of your body into one of two categories: your fat mass and everything else. What isn't fat mass is considered lean body mass, which consists of your bones, muscles, hair, and water.

HIIT is scientifically proven to burn body fat as well as generating lean muscle. Because muscle weighs more than fat, just tracking your weight may be a poor indication of your progress when undertaking HIIT. Knowing your body fat percentage can help you determine realistic goals, but keep in mind that it is just one of many ways to set goals and measure your fitness. For most people, the ultimate goal is to have a better-looking, healthier body. Don't become obsessed with body fat percentage or any other measurement.

There are many different methods for measuring body fat, some more accurate than others. I advocate using a tape measure and the military method, which is the formula used by the U.S. Department of Defense for measuring body fat percentage.

GET YOUR MEASUREMENTS

Use a tape measure to record the circumference of your neck, waist, and hips. Measure in inches or centimeters.

Neck. Measure neck circumference at a point just below the larynx (Adam's apple) and perpendicular to the long axis of the neck. Round the measurement up to the nearest half inch (or half centimeter).

Waist. Measure the natural waist circumference, against the skin, at the narrowest point of the abdomen. This is usually about halfway between the navel and the lower end of the sternum (breast bone). Be sure the tape is level and parallel to the floor. Round the measurement down to the nearest half inch (or half centimeter).

Hip. Measure the hip circumference, passing the measuring tape over the greatest protrusion of the glutes as viewed from the side. Make sure the tape is level and parallel to the floor. Round the hip measurement down to the nearest half inch (or half centimeter).

You will also need to know your height in inches or centimeters.

CALCULATE YOUR BODY FAT

To calculate your body fat percentage, plug your measurements into an online calculator: corepilatesandfitness.com/page18/index.html
You can also find your body fat percentage using the following formulas and a calculator with the LOG function.

For measurements in inches:
Body fat percentage = 163.205 × LOG(abdomen + hip - neck) - 97.684 × LOG(height) - 78.387

For measurements in centimeters:
Body fat percentage = 163.205 × LOG(abdomen + hip - neck) - 97.684 × LOG(height) - 104.912

The America Council on Exercise provides the following guidelines for body fat percentage in women.
31 or higher: obese
25–31: acceptable
21–24: fit
14–20: athletic
Less than 13: essential fat levels

SET YOUR GOALS

Developing sound goals is critical to your performance. If you want to see long-term, sustainable success, then you need to be clear about what you want to accomplish.

BE SMART

Successful goal setting requires SMART goals. Keep this acronym in mind when you consider what you want to achieve.

SMART GOALS ARE...

Specific: Goals should be simple and clearly define what you are going to do.

Example: "To perform 20 push-ups in 30 seconds."

Measurable: Goals should be measurable, providing tangible evidence that you have met your goal.

Example: "To lose 10 pounds in six weeks." This is measurable. In six weeks, you will either have met your goal or not. The goal "to lose weight" is not measurable.

Achievable: Goals need to be both challenging and realistic.

Example: "To lose 50 pounds in six weeks" is not achievable or realistic. Losing 10 pounds in six weeks would be realistic, healthy, and sustainable.

Results-driven: Goals should be relevant and measure outcomes, not activities.

Example: "Go to the gym" is an activity. "Burn 500 calories doing HIIT at the gym" is results driven.

Time-bound: Goals should be linked to a time frame that creates a practical sense of urgency. Give yourself a deadline.

Example: "I want to lose 10 pounds in six weeks," not "I want to lose 10 pounds."

STICK TO YOUR GOALS

Making your goals is just the first step. Now you have to stick to them. It's not easy, but there are a few strategies that can help you stay on track.

1 Write them down.

Studies show writing a goal down leads to a greater percentage of completion. Twice a year I take stock of my life, sit down, and type up a goal sheet. I have them posted on my bathroom mirror, in a frame on my desk at work, and even stuck to the front of the fridge. The more you see your goals, the greater the chance that you'll achieve them.

2 Be specific.

If you've created SMART goals, you should have this one covered. Goals are most often achieved when they are tangible, measurable, and specific. For example, you might set a time goal for running a race or target a specific body fat percentage.

3 Share them with the world.

Studies show that people are more accountable when they believe others expect them to do something. Share your fitness goals on Facebook, post them on Twitter, tell your significant other, and alert your friends. Take pride in your goals and don't be afraid to ask others for their support and motivation. When you successfully meet those goals, share that, too!

4 Take small bites.

Give yourself the chance to feel a sense of achievement. Take your larger goal and divide it into smaller steps. At the completion of each step, take a moment to enjoy that success. It will help motivate you to achieve the next step.

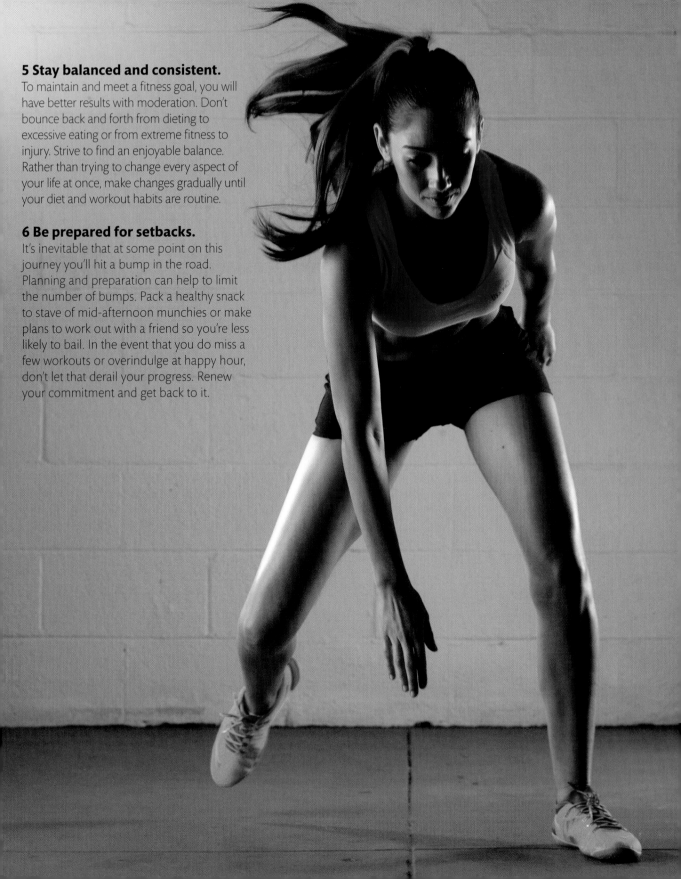

5 Stay balanced and consistent.
To maintain and meet a fitness goal, you will
have better results with moderation. Don't
bounce back and forth from dieting to
excessive eating or from extreme fitness to
injury. Strive to find an enjoyable balance.
Rather than trying to change every aspect of
your life at once, make changes gradually until
your diet and workout habits are routine.

6 Be prepared for setbacks.
It's inevitable that at some point on this
journey you'll hit a bump in the road.
Planning and preparation can help to limit
the number of bumps. Pack a healthy snack
to stave of mid-afternoon munchies or make
plans to work out with a friend so you're less
likely to bail. In the event that you do miss a
few workouts or overindulge at happy hour,
don't let that derail your progress. Renew
your commitment and get back to it.

RECOVERY

When you're pushing yourself to the limit during your workout, you need to allow time for rest and recovery. Recovery is critical for injury prevention and consistent training, and it enables you to give maximal effort every time you open this book and take on one of the routines.

HYDRATION AND NUTRITION

Keeping your body properly fueled will aid in recovery. Replace your fluids and electrolytes to prevent dehydration, and be sure to get enough protein and carbohydrates to rebuild muscle tissue and stay energized.

TRAINER TIP

Two products that I recommend for recovery are SOS Rehydrate (sosrehydrate.com) and Frog Fuel (frogperformance.com). SOS Rehydrate delivers the electrolytes you need with only 25 calories per serving. Frog Fuel is an excellent, portable source of protein and amino acids that your body can quickly absorb.

USING A FOAM ROLLER

A key component of recovery is self-myofascial release using a foam roller. The fascia is connective tissue that wraps around the muscles in the body. This tissue can become tense or constricted while working out, causing pain.

Using a foam roller to "roll out" the muscles can alleviate soreness and stiffness, promote circulation of oxygenated blood, and even break up scar tissue and restrictions in the fascia. A foam roller also allows you to apply targeted pressure to specific spots in the muscle that may be causing pain.

I recommend using a three-inch high-density foam roller. These can easily be found at sporting goods stores or online.

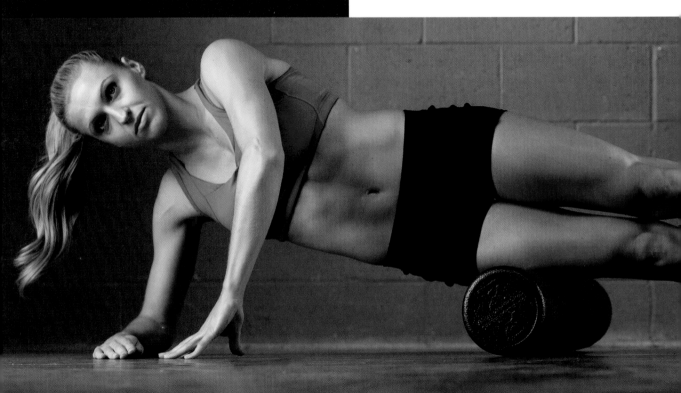

FOAM ROLLING TECHNIQUE

The foam roller can be used on many parts of the body, including the legs, back, and arms. Regardless of the area you're targeting, the basic technique is the same. Use the roller as a warm-up, after working out, or whenever you feel pain.

1 Position your body on the roller. The weight of your body will apply pressure on your muscles. Roll back and forth slowly. When you find a tender spot in the area you are working, pause and wait for the discomfort to diminish. This could take up to one minute and may be uncomfortable.

2 When the area is no longer sensitive, begin to roll up and down the muscle on the roller. Identify any other sensitive spots and repeat.

3 When tender areas can be rolled over without pain, continue rolling regularly to keep the area relaxed. There is a lot of freedom for experimentation and "feel" when using the roller. See what works best for you and manipulate the roller to the correct position. You can create your own techniques to meet your needs.

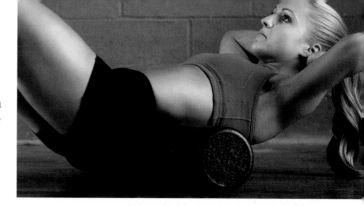

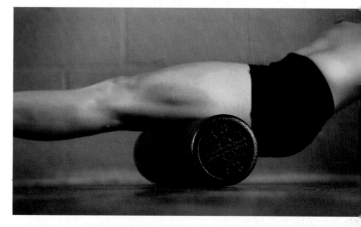

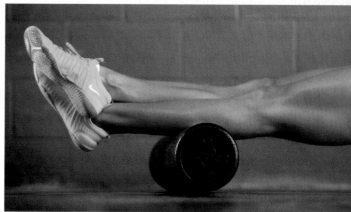

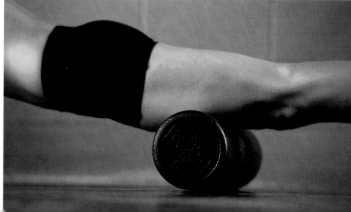

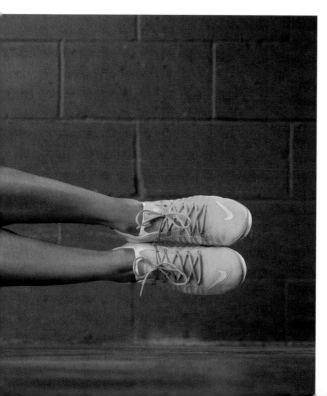

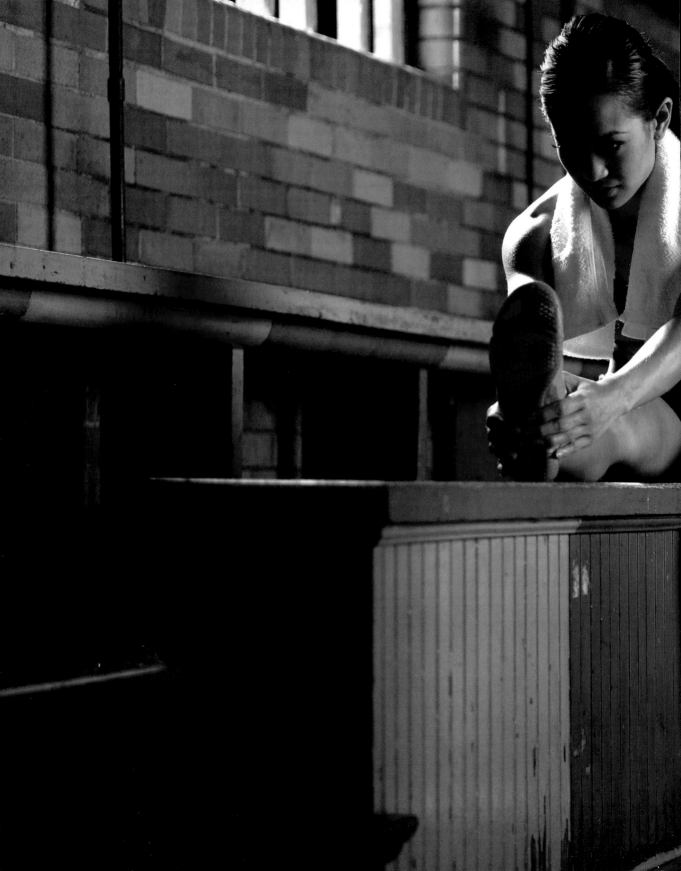

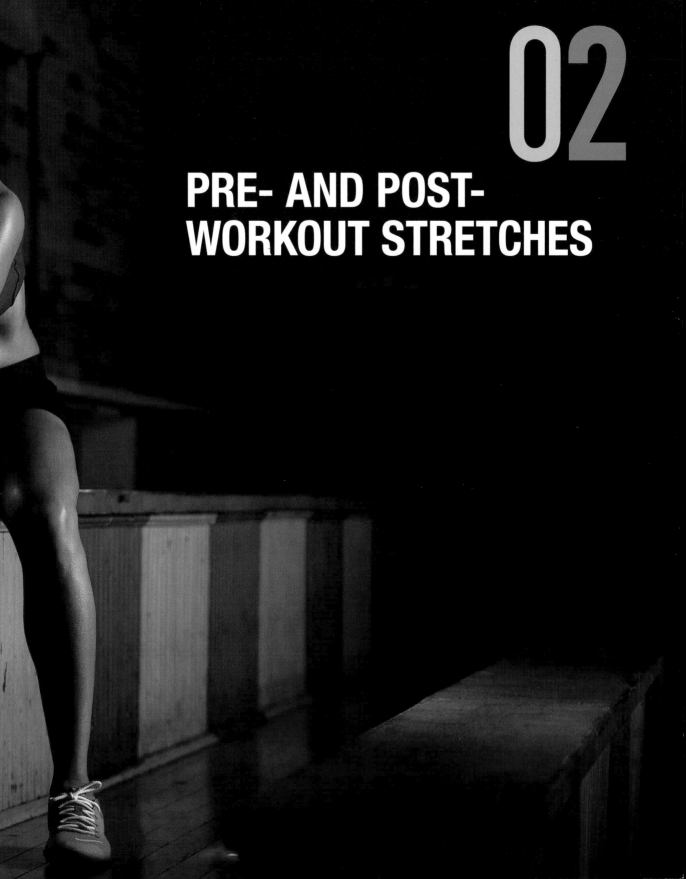

PRE- AND POST-WORKOUT STRETCHES

02

FORWARD FOLD TO FLAT BACK FOLD

A staple in yoga classes, the forward fold, or *uttanasana*, stretches the hamstrings and calves and releases the low back. By developing the forward fold into flat back fold, or *ardha uttanasana*, you can increase the stretch to include the hips. This stretch will increase flexibility and prevent injury.

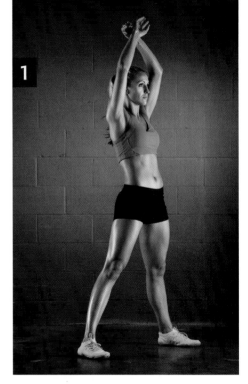

Stand tall with arms loosely by your sides. Inhale and lift arms overhead.

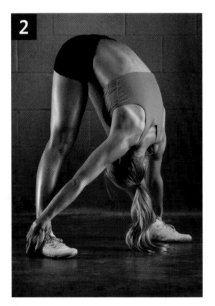

Exhale and release arms down either side of your body. Bend forward from the hips and roll down your spine, bringing your nose toward your shins.

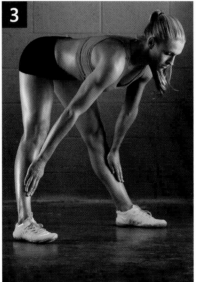

Inhale and lift your head as you flatten your back and shift your weight back, lifting your butt. Place hands as far up on the legs as needed to comfortably flatten your back.

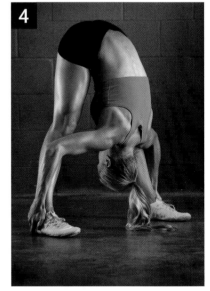

Exhale and return to your forward fold. Repeat three times.

SIDE LUNGE

The side lunge is a dynamic stretch that tones and stretches the lower body, building strength at the same time. The side lunge opens the hips, creating stability and balance. It also stretches the hips, calves, Achilles tendons, hamstrings, and groin. It combines the components and benefits of three popular yoga poses: low crescent lunge, chair pose, and side angle pose.

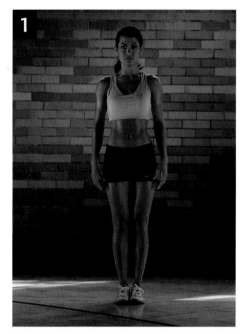

Stand tall, feet together, and hands hanging loosely at your sides.

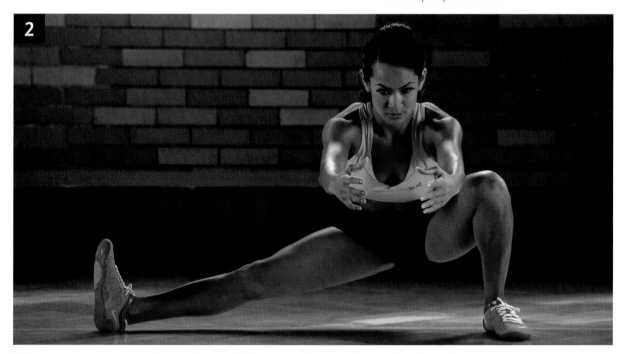

Take a giant step to your right. Bend your right knee to at least 90 degrees, but lower if possible. Extend your arms in front of you for balance. Hold for approximately 30 seconds before returning to center. Repeat three times on each side.

DEEP LUNGE STRETCH

Tight hip flexors can inhibit your abs, glutes, and inner thighs from getting the results you want from your workouts. They can also cause injuries, including lower back pain, IT band syndrome, and even pattelar tendonitis. The deep lunge is an activation stretch that will wake up and stretch the hip flexors, making your workouts more efficient and preventing injury.

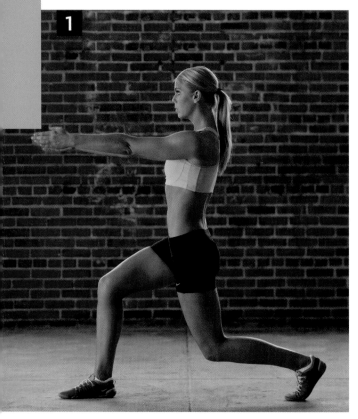

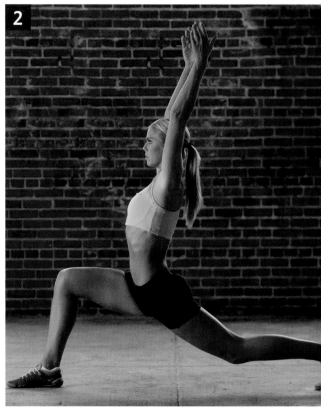

Lunge forward with your right leg, keeping your knee bent at 90 degrees and your weight in your heel. Your left knee should be bent under your hip. Raise your arms until they are parallel to the floor and make sure your toes are pointing forward.

Reach your hands toward the ceiling, keeping your arms in line with your ears. Extend the back leg and sink your hips down slightly. Hold for two to three deep breaths. Return to start and repeat five times before switching to the left leg.

EXTENDED SIDE ANGLE POSE

Extended side angle pose is a popular yoga posture that strengthens your thighs, hips, and ankles while stretching your groin, back, and hips and opening the chest. This stretch can also increase lung capacity.

TRAINER TIP
If your hands do not comfortably reach the floor, place a yoga brick or something similar under the supporting hand.

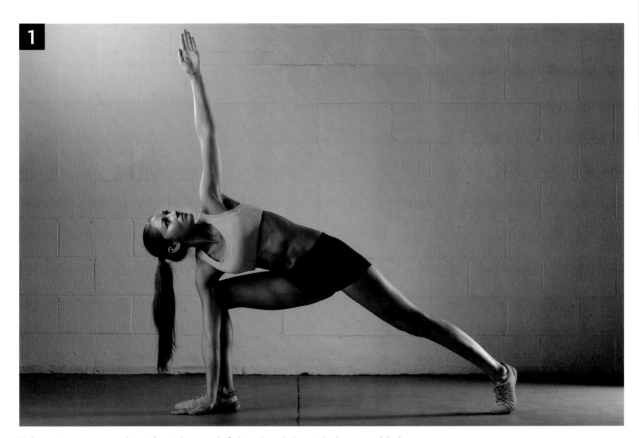

Take a giant step to the side with your left leg. Bend the right knee to 90 degrees so that the thigh is parallel to the floor. Bring the right hand to the floor and extend the left arm to the ceiling, opening your chest. Hold for 30 seconds and repeat on the opposite side.

TRIANGLE FORWARD FOLD

The triangle forward fold is an asymmetrical standing forward bend called *parsvottanasana* in yoga. It is an excellent way to stretch and activate the hamstrings while protecting the lower back.

TRAINER TIP

Keep a soft bend in the knee of the front leg to avoid unnecessary pressure on the joint and ligaments. If needed, place your hands on the shin of your front leg for added stability.

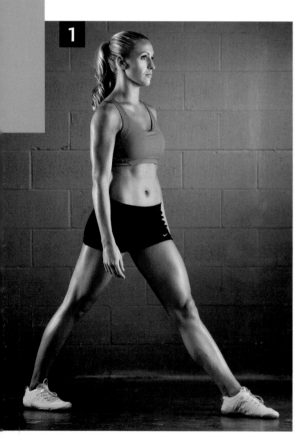

Stand tall, feet wider than shoulders with arms loosely hanging by sides. Take a giant step forward with the left foot. Keep the toes of both feet pointing forward.

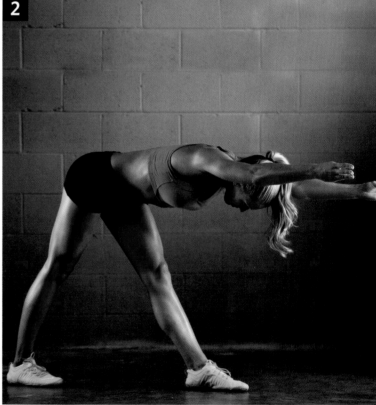

Bend slowly from the hips, keeping your spine as long as possible. Pull the right hip forward to square the pelvis and reach out with the arms, activating the hamstrings to keep the torso horizontal. Hold for 30 seconds and take 5 to 10 deep breaths. Repeat on the opposite side.

HIP OPENER

Opening the hips can have many benefits; easing back pain, improving your gait, and even improving circulation in the legs. The hip opener stretches the groin, lower back, base of the spine, and hips. By releasing the muscles of the hips (the psoas major and illiacus), you can prevent injury and boost athletic performance.

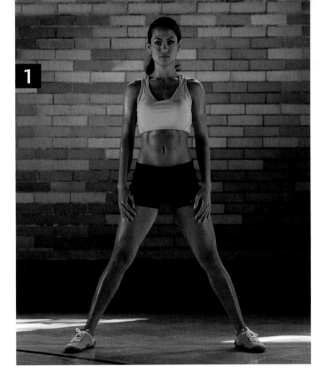

Stand tall, with feet wider than shoulders and arms loosely hanging by sides. Turn your feet out, opening your hips.

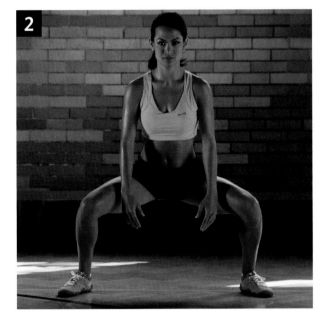

Bend at the knees, lowering hips toward the floor. Try to get as deep as you can while maintaining a long spine. Keep your knees directly over your toes; don't allow them to buckle inward.

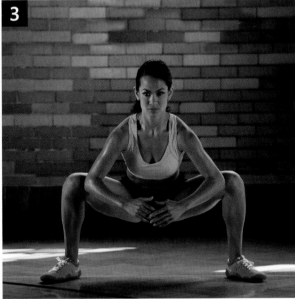

Bring your elbows to the insides of your thighs and gently press them out. Hold for approximately 30 seconds while you take long, deep breaths. Repeat three times.

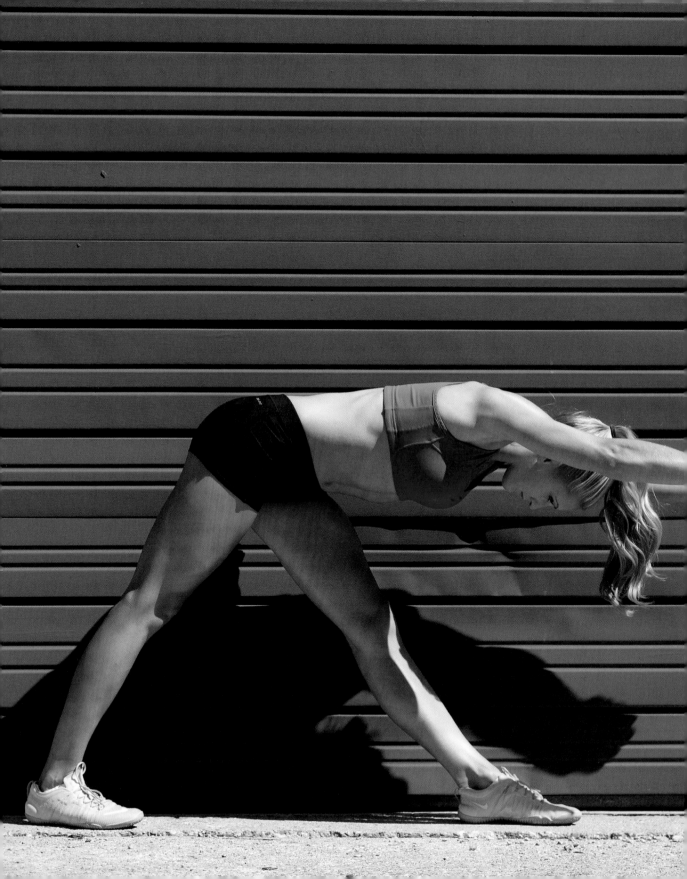

03

INTRODUCTORY
HIIT ROUTINES

LEVEL 1:
INTRODUCTORY ROUTINES

These five introductory routines are designed to get you started with HIIT by introducing base exercises and common routine formats in a way that is varied and challenging without being overwhelming. Level 1 will get things rolling with lower impact exercises, shorter routines, and longer rest periods. Remember the golden rule during each of these routines: form first and speed second.

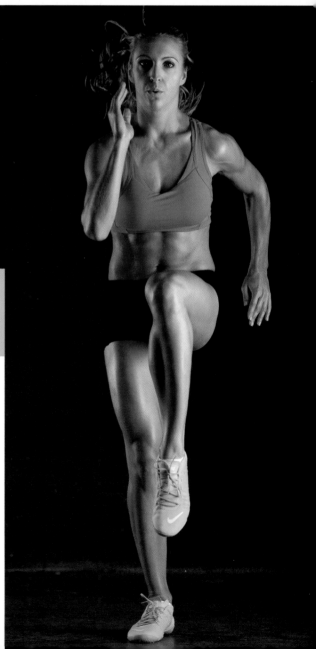

EASY DOES HIIT
TOTAL TIME: 9:00

These four classic and simple HIIT exercises provide a total body workout at a 2:1 work-to-rest ratio, which means you'll be working for twice as long as you rest. Push hard, have fun, and let's HIIT IT!

Repeat the set three times.
Rest for one minute after each set.

TRAINER TIP
For both squats and push-ups, depth is far more important than speed. If you need to, perform the push-ups from your knees.

	WORK	REST
SPRINT	0:20	0:10
SQUAT	0:20	0:10
JUMPING JACK	0:20	0:10
PUSH-UP	0:20	0:10

THE FAB FOUR

TOTAL TIME: 7:30

The second routine in the Level 1 introductory series acquaints you with the 4:1 work-to-rest ratio, meaning your work time is four times as long as your rest time. The 4:1 work-to-rest ratio is used frequently across all levels because it challenges you to work at your maximal heart rate for a short but intense burst.

Repeat the set three times.
Rest for 30 seconds after each set.

	WORK	REST
HIGH KNEES	0:30	0:00
SKI JUMP	0:30	0:00
SEAL JACK	0:30	0:00
PLANK	0:30	0:00

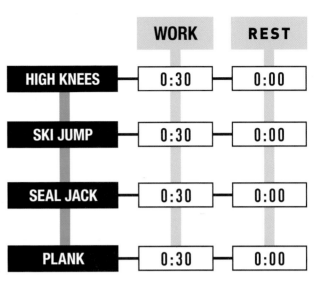

TRAINER TIP

When performing ski jumps, be sure to land softly. Keep your hips facing forward and bend at the hips, knees, and ankles to absorb the impact of landing and decelerate your body.

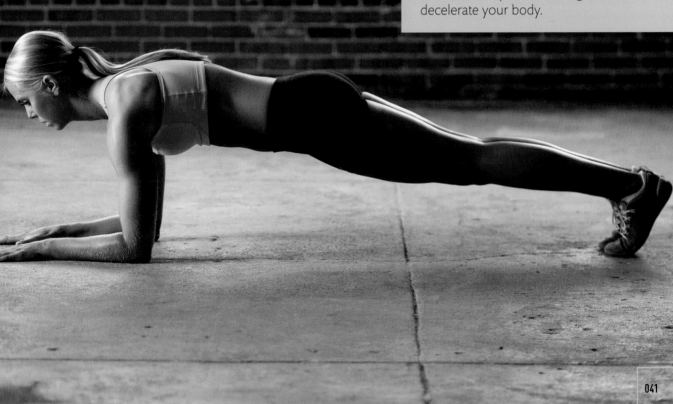

ENDURO

TOTAL TIME: 10:00

The third Level 1 introductory routine will familiarize you with the longer cardiovascular- and muscular endurance-oriented routines. These are especially beneficial if you play sports that require sustained activity for long periods of time.

Repeat the set two times.
Rest one minute after each set.

TRAINER TIP

If working for four minutes at high intensity with no break is too much for you, try adding a 10-second rest after each exercise.

	WORK	REST
SPRINT	0:30	0:00
SQUAT	0:30	0:00
SEAL JACK	0:30	0:00
PUSH-UP	0:30	0:00
HIGH KNEES	0:30	0:00
REVERSE LUNGE	0:30	0:00
THE MUMMY	0:30	0:00
PLANK	0:30	0:00

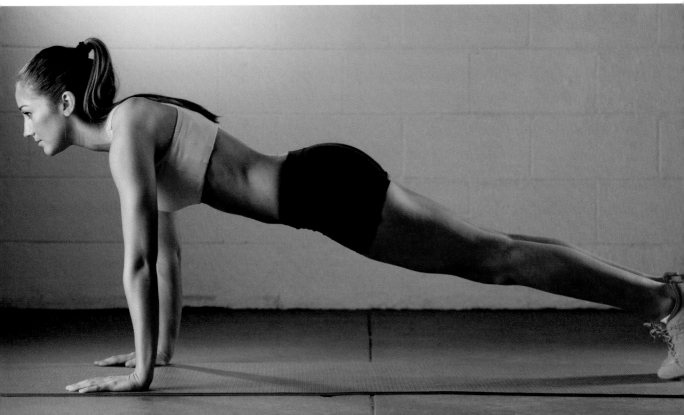

EVERY SECOND COUNTS

TOTAL TIME: 12:00

Every second counts in the fourth introductory routine for Level 1. This pyramid format routine has a decreasing rest period by round; the more tired you become, the less recovery time you get. Compound multi-muscle exercises and an increasing cardiovascular challenge make this as tough physically as it is mentally.

Complete all three rounds in order. Rest one minute after each round.

TRAINER TIP
Focus on quality, not quantity. As you get tired, pay close attention to your form to prevent injury.

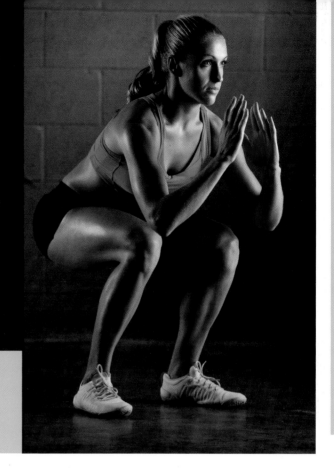

	ROUND 1 WORK / REST	ROUND 2 WORK / REST	ROUND 3 WORK / REST
JUMPING JACK	0:15 / 0:15	0:20 / 0:10	0:30 / 0:00
LATERAL LUNGE	0:15 / 0:15	0:20 / 0:10	0:30 / 0:00
MOUNTAIN CLIMBER	0:15 / 0:15	0:20 / 0:10	0:30 / 0:00
X-JACK	0:15 / 0:15	0:20 / 0:10	0:30 / 0:00
SQUAT HOLD	0:15 / 0:15	0:20 / 0:10	0:30 / 0:00
PUSH-UP	0:15 / 0:15	0:20 / 0:10	0:30 / 0:00

THREE-PEAT

TOTAL TIME: 27:00

Three is the magic number in the final introductory routine to Level 1. You'll do each three-minute set three times, making this the longest of the Level 1 introductory routines.

Do each set three times. Rest for one minute after each set.

CHALLENGE

If you're not feeling challenged, drop the rest time down to 30 seconds between sets.

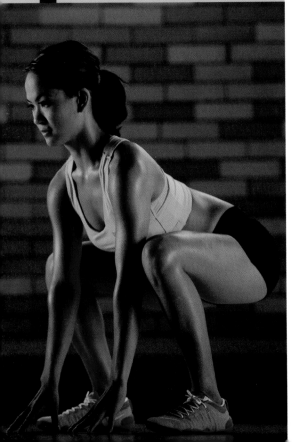

SET 1	WORK	REST
HIGH KNEES	0:30	0:00
SEAL JACK	0:30	0:00
SPRINT	0:30	0:00
CROSS JACK	0:30	0:00

SET 2	WORK	REST
SQUAT	0:30	0:00
REVERSE LUNGE	0:30	0:00
SQUAT LIFT (RIGHT)	0:30	0:00
SQUAT LIFT (LEFT)	0:30	0:00

SET 3	WORK	REST
THE MUMMY	0:30	0:00
PUSH-UP	0:30	0:00
BICYCLE CRUNCH	0:30	0:00
PLANK	0:30	0:00

LEVEL 2:
INTRODUCTORY ROUTINES

The five Level 2 introductory routines focus on HIIT basics in a variety of routine formats. These routines are more challenging than those for Level 1 and include plyometrics (jump training), frequent elevation changes, and an increased level of difficulty. It's time to raise the bar!

HIIT ME AGAIN

TOTAL TIME: 9:00

The first routine for Level 2 incorporates explosive movements and multiplanar exercises. The challenge gets dialed up a notch so you will have to dig a little deeper and work a little harder.

Repeat the set three times.
Rest for one minute after each set.

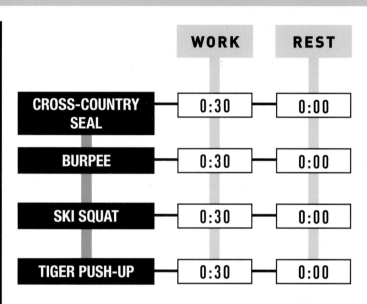

	WORK	REST
CROSS-COUNTRY SEAL	0:30	0:00
BURPEE	0:30	0:00
SKI SQUAT	0:30	0:00
TIGER PUSH-UP	0:30	0:00

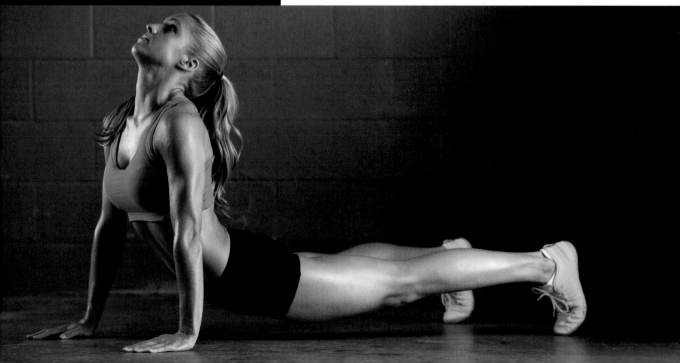

JUMP UP AND GET DOWN

TOTAL TIME: 8:00

The second introductory routine for Level 2 focuses on plyometrics, or jumping exercises. These exercises require muscles to be repeatedly and rapidly stretched (loaded) and then contracted. This rapid stretching and contracting increases muscular power and mimics the movements used in many sports. Get familiar with plyometric exercises to increase agility, balance, coordination, and athletic performance. Now jump to it!

Repeat the set two times.
Rest for 30 seconds after each set.

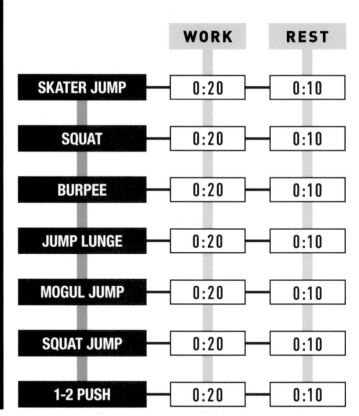

	WORK	REST
SKATER JUMP	0:20	0:10
SQUAT	0:20	0:10
BURPEE	0:20	0:10
JUMP LUNGE	0:20	0:10
MOGUL JUMP	0:20	0:10
SQUAT JUMP	0:20	0:10
1-2 PUSH	0:20	0:10

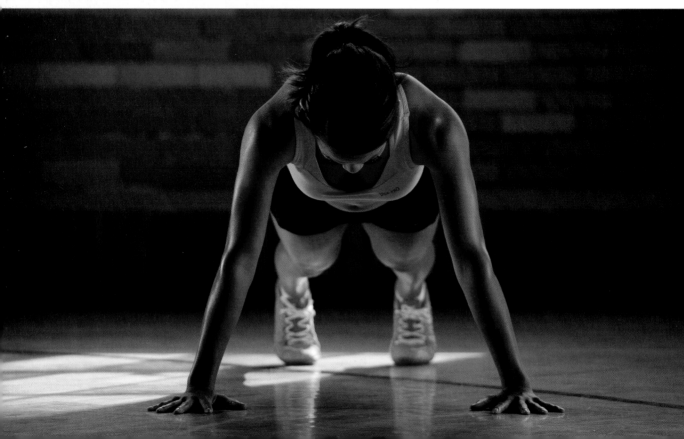

SORE OR SORRY?

TOTAL TIME: 5:00

Will you wake up tomorrow sore but satisfied, or sorry that you didn't work out? The third introductory routine for Level 2 gets you familiar with the 4:1 work-to-rest ratio that is often used for HIIT routines. With this ratio, the length of time you work is four times the length of your rest.

Do each set twice. Rest for 30 seconds after each set.

SET 1	WORK	REST
SPRINT	0:30	0:00
GRASSHOPPER	0:30	0:00
X-JACK	0:30	0:00
MOUNTAIN CLIMBER	0:30	0:00

SET 2	WORK	REST
SQUAT	0:30	0:00
REVERSE LUNGE	0:30	0:00
SQUAT JUMP	0:30	0:00
JUMP LUNGE	0:30	0:00

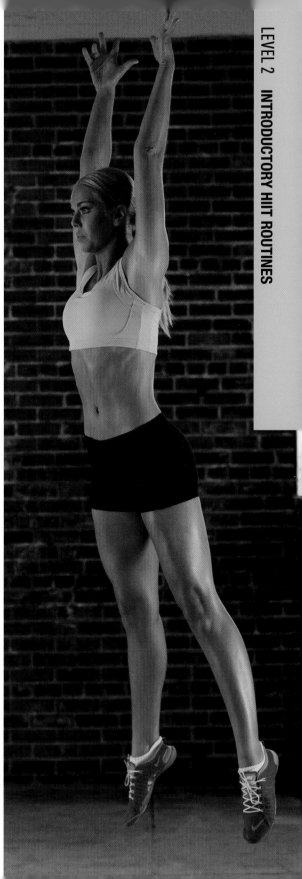

IN HIIT TO WIN IT

TOTAL TIME: 14:00

The fourth routine in the Level 2 introductory series bumps it up a notch with eight total-body exercises engineered to firm and burn. Push as hard as possible; maximal effort equals maximal results.

**Repeat the set two times.
Rest for one minute after each set.**

	WORK	REST
SPRINT	0:30	0:15
SKATER JUMP	0:30	0:15
SQUAT PEDAL	0:30	0:15
SIDE SUICIDES	0:30	0:15
1-2 PUSH	0:30	0:15
LATERAL LUNGE	0:30	0:15
CROSS PUSH	0:30	0:15
SPRINTER SIT-UP	0:30	0:15

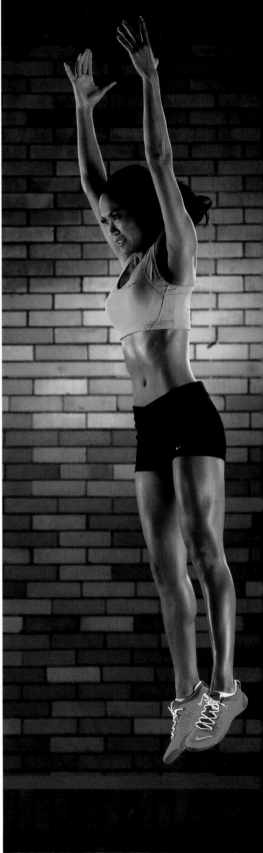

SET 1	WORK	REST
JUMPING JACK	0:30	0:00
SQUAT JUMP	0:30	0:00
SIDE SUICIDES	0:30	0:00
JUMP LUNGE	0:30	0:00

SET 2	WORK	REST
SPRINT	0:30	0:00
T-STAND (RIGHT)	0:30	0:00
BURPEE	0:30	0:00
T-STAND (LEFT)	0:30	0:00

SET 3	WORK	REST
V-UP	0:30	0:00
1-2 PUSH	0:30	0:00
SPRINTER SIT-UP	0:30	0:00
PLANK PUNCH	0:30	0:00

KEEP HIIT MOVING!

TOTAL TIME: 22:30

The final and longest routine in the Level 2 introductory series, this workout will tone, tighten, and strengthen—and give you a glimpse of what awaits in Level 3.

Do each set three times. Rest for 30 seconds after each set.

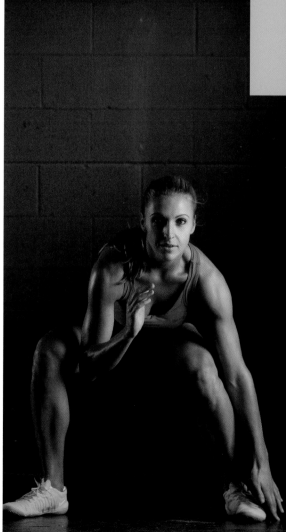

LEVEL 3:
INTRODUCTORY ROUTINES

Level 3 is all about maximal output. The five Level 3 introductory routines will get you familiar with HIIT while providing a challenging workout. This level features the most difficult exercises and the least amount of recovery time, making you really earn your results.

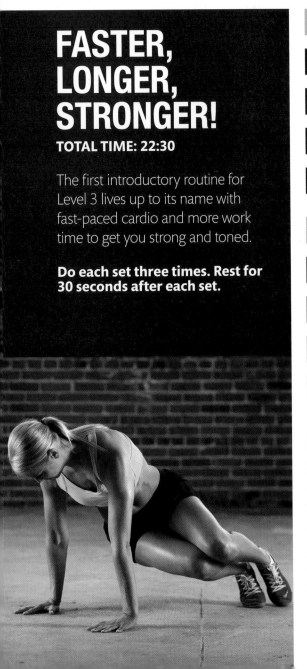

FASTER, LONGER, STRONGER!

TOTAL TIME: 22:30

The first introductory routine for Level 3 lives up to its name with fast-paced cardio and more work time to get you strong and toned.

Do each set three times. Rest for 30 seconds after each set.

SET 1	WORK	REST
SPRINT	0:30	0:00
X-JACK	0:30	0:00
SKI SQUAT	0:30	0:00
CRAB TOUCH	0:30	0:00

SET 2	WORK	REST
POWER KNEE (RIGHT)	0:30	0:00
IN AND OUT	0:30	0:00
POWER KNEE (LEFT)	0:30	0:00
SPIDERMAN	0:30	0:00

SET 3	WORK	REST
BURPEE	0:30	0:00
SIDE SUICIDES	0:30	0:00
SQUAT PEDAL	0:30	0:00
1-2 PUSH	0:30	0:00

POWER OF THREE

TOTAL TIME: 22:30

As the Level 3 routines get harder and the exercises become more complex, it's imperative to pay attention to your form. Push as hard as you can, but focus on quality over quantity.

Do each set three times. Rest for 30 seconds after each set.

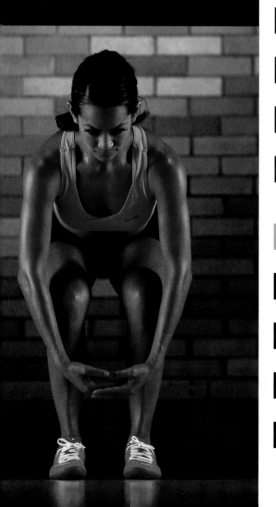

SET 1	WORK	REST
JUMPING JACK	0:30	0:00
MOUNTAIN CLIMBER	0:30	0:00
MOGUL JUMP	0:30	0:00
STAR	0:30	0:00

SET 2	WORK	REST
SQUAT JUMP	0:30	0:00
SQUAT HOLD	0:30	0:00
JUMP LUNGE	0:30	0:00
SQUAT HOLD	0:30	0:00

SET 3	WORK	REST
TIGER PUSH-UP	0:30	0:00
REACH	0:30	0:00
V-UP	0:30	0:00
RUSSIAN TWIST	0:30	0:00

FIERCELY FIT

TOTAL TIME: 15:00

The third routine in the Level 3 introductory series keeps you working hard with eight exercises selected to build core strength and tone your legs. The 4:1 work-to-rest ratio will kick your heart rate into high gear.

Repeat the set three times.
Rest for one minute after each set.

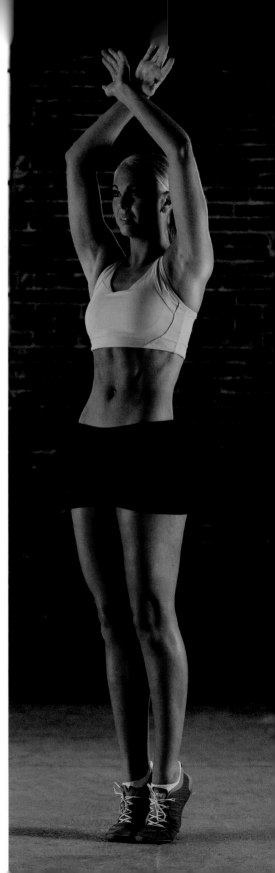

	WORK	REST
SPRINT	0:30	0:00
JUMP LUNGE	0:30	0:00
GRASSHOPPER	0:30	0:00
STAR	0:30	0:00
SQUAT JUMP	0:30	0:00
BALL PRESS	0:30	0:00
ALTERNATING LEG LIFT BURPEE	0:30	0:00
PLANK ROTATION	0:30	0:00

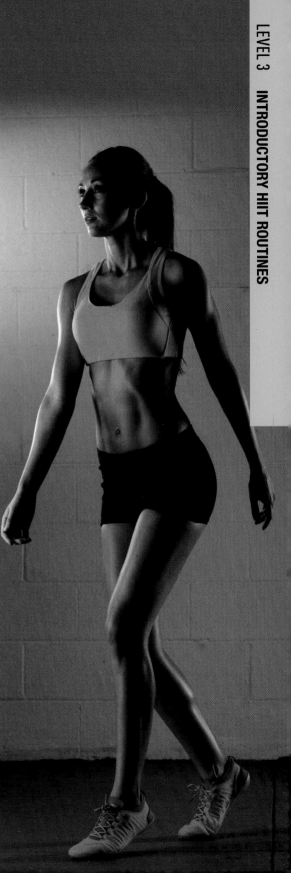

CUT TO THE CORE

TOTAL TIME: 15:00

The fourth Level 3 introductory routine features a combination of cardio and upper body work at a 4:1 work-to-rest ratio. Push yourself as hard as you can, even on round three.

Repeat the set three times.
Rest for one minute after each set.

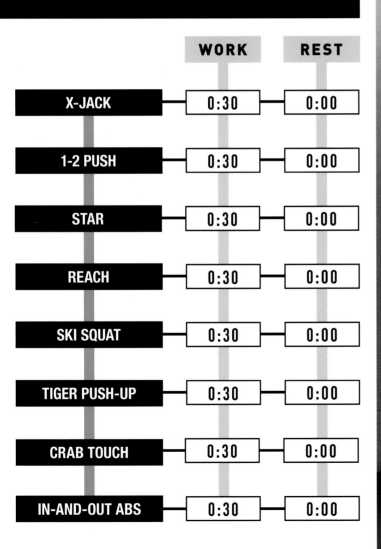

	WORK	REST
X-JACK	0:30	0:00
1-2 PUSH	0:30	0:00
STAR	0:30	0:00
REACH	0:30	0:00
SKI SQUAT	0:30	0:00
TIGER PUSH-UP	0:30	0:00
CRAB TOUCH	0:30	0:00
IN-AND-OUT ABS	0:30	0:00

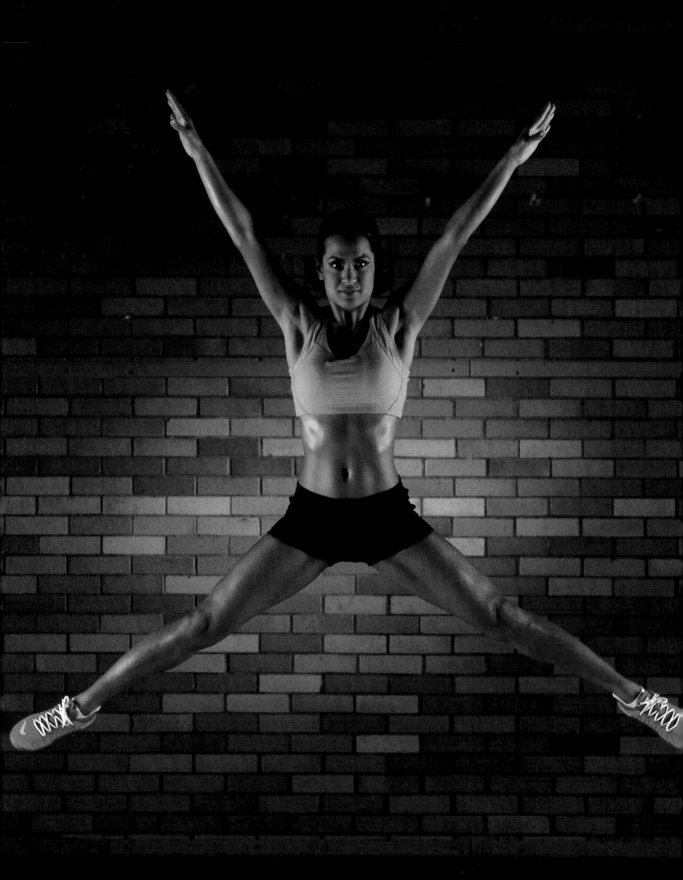

FINAL COUNTDOWN

TOTAL TIME: 40:00

The last of the Level 3 introductory routines builds endurance with four intense compound sets to keep your body on its toes, incinerate calories, and prepare you for the wide variety of HIIT challenges to come.

**Do Set 1 one time. Do Sets 2 to 4 three times each.
Rest for one minute after each set.**

SET 1 (1 ROUND)

	WORK	REST
X-JACK	0:30	0:00
1-2 PUSH	0:30	0:00
STAR	0:30	0:00
REACH	0:30	0:00
SKI SQUAT	0:30	0:00
TIGER PUSH-UP	0:30	0:00
CRAB TOUCH	0:30	0:00
IN-AND-OUT ABS	0:30	0:00

SET 2 (3 ROUNDS)

	WORK	REST
JUMPING JACK	0:30	0:00
MOUNTAIN CLIMBER	0:30	0:00
MOGUL JUMP	0:30	0:00
LATERAL LUNGE	0:30	0:00

SET 3 (3 ROUNDS)

	WORK	REST
SQUAT JUMP	0:30	0:00
SQUAT HOLD	0:30	0:00
PEDAL	0:30	0:00
SQUAT HOLD	0:30	0:00

SET 4 (3 ROUNDS)

	WORK	REST
PUSH-UP	0:30	0:00
TRICEP DIP	0:30	0:00
V-UP	0:30	0:00
RUSSIAN TWIST	0:30	0:00

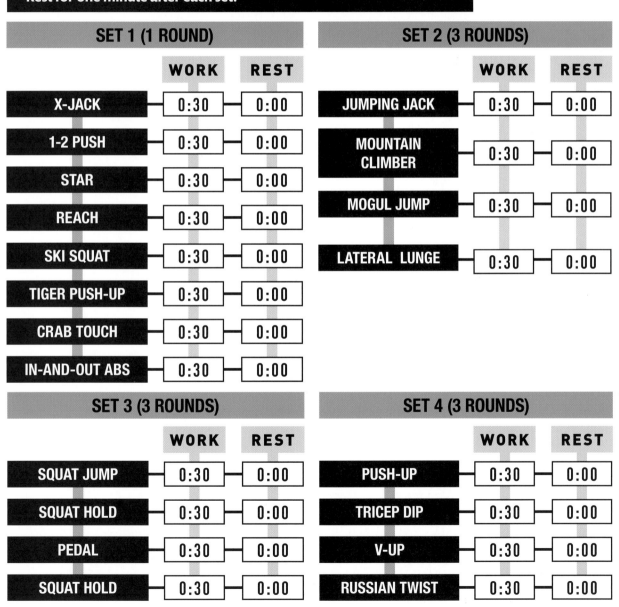

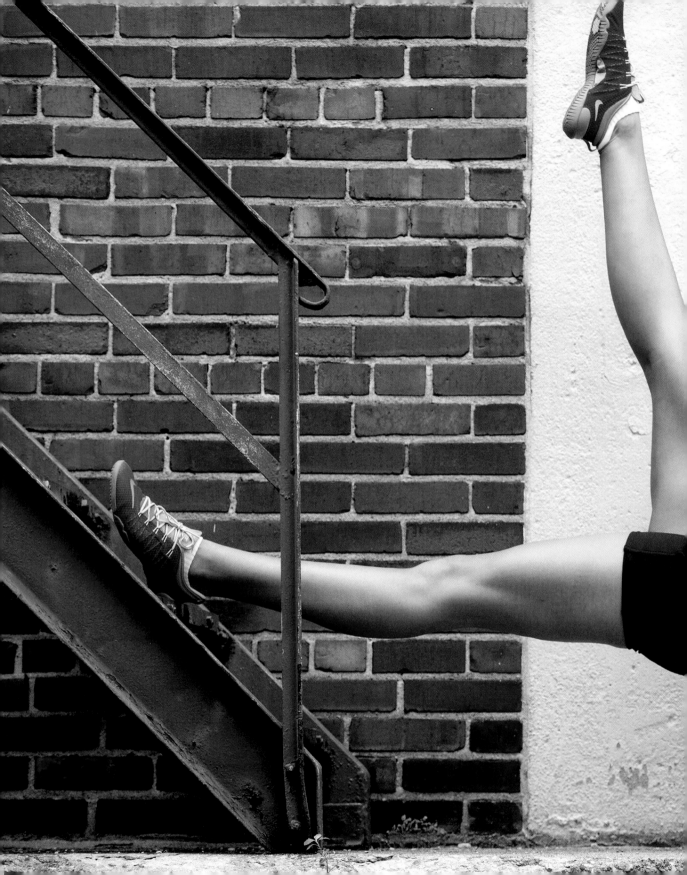

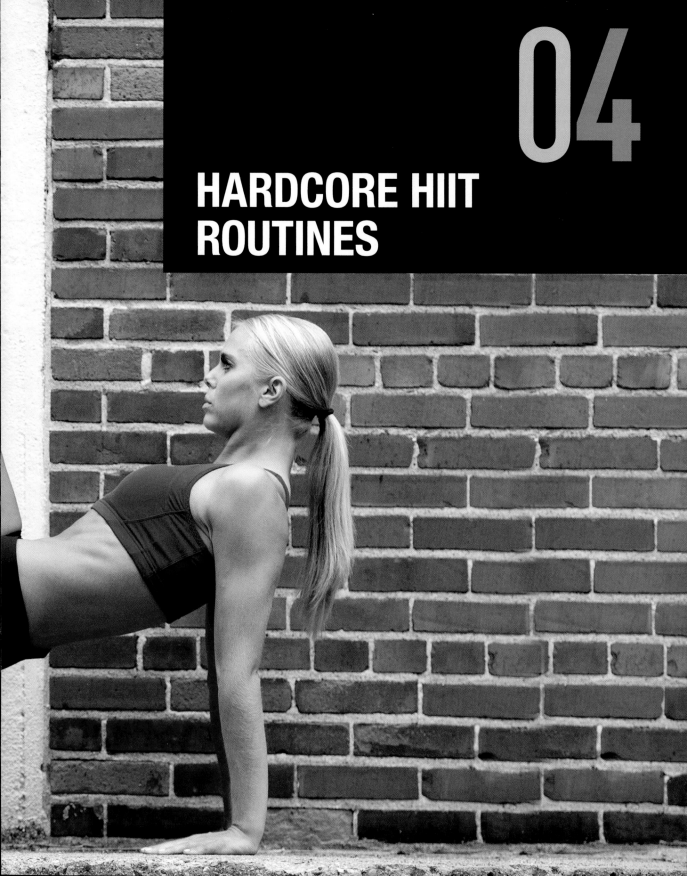

04

HARDCORE HIIT ROUTINES

JUST DO HIIT!

This simple, fun, and sweaty routine brings together three HIIT basics: sprints, squats, and burpees. Push for maximum heart rate, and remember: you get out what you put in. Good Luck!

Rest for one minute between each round.

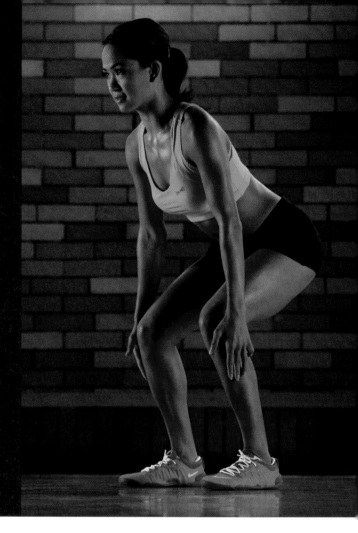

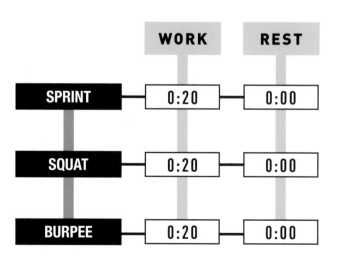

	WORK	REST
SPRINT	0:20	0:00
SQUAT	0:20	0:00
BURPEE	0:20	0:00

LEVEL 1 - 4 ROUNDS
TOTAL TIME: 8:00

LEVEL 2 - 8 ROUNDS
TOTAL TIME: 16:00

LEVEL 3 - 12 ROUNDS
TOTAL TIME: 24:00

LEG HELL

This workout pushes your legs to the limit with a series of exercises targeting your calves, hamstrings, and glutes. Your legs will never be stronger, tighter, or more defined. At a 4:1 work-to-rest ratio, it won't be easy, but it will be worth it!

Rest for 30 seconds between each round.

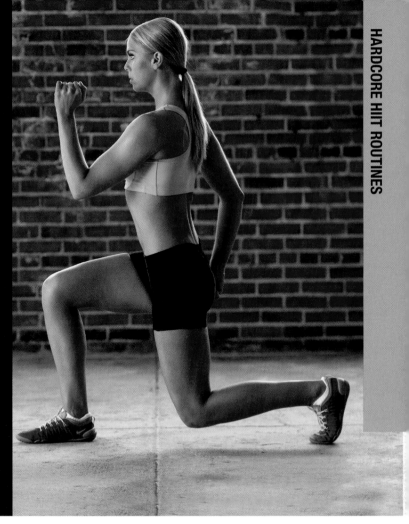

	WORK	REST
SQUAT	0:30	0:00
REVERSE LUNGE	0:30	0:00
JUMP LUNGE	0:30	0:00
SQUAT JUMP	0:30	0:00

LEVEL 1 - 2 ROUNDS
TOTAL TIME: 5:00

LEVEL 2 - 3 ROUNDS
TOTAL TIME: 7:30

LEVEL 3 - 4 ROUNDS
TOTAL TIME: 10:00

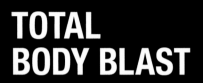

TOTAL BODY BLAST

This routine includes some of the most common compound (multi-muscle) exercises. By working multiple large muscle groups in unison, you stoke the body's fat-burning furnace, incinerating calories and creating muscle tone, definition, and strength in the process.

For all levels, do one set.

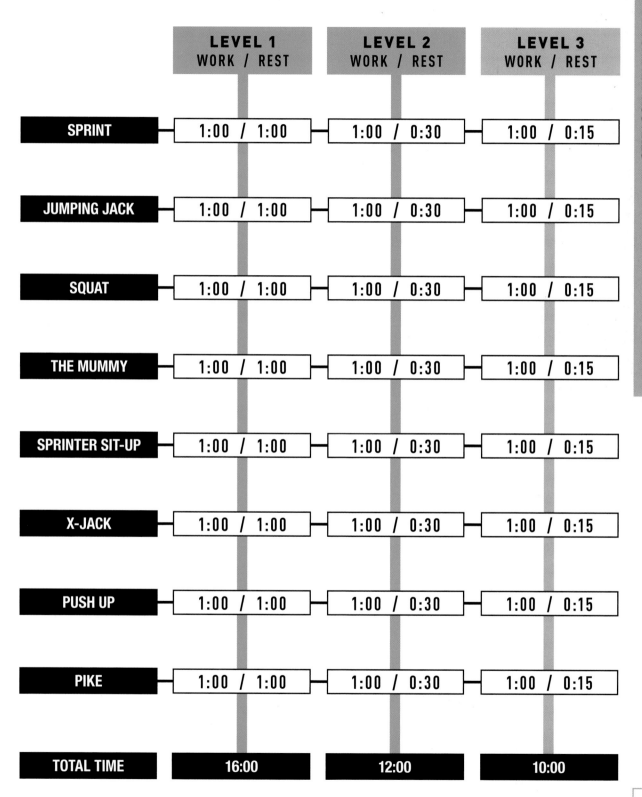

	LEVEL 1 WORK / REST	LEVEL 2 WORK / REST	LEVEL 3 WORK / REST
SPRINT	1:00 / 1:00	1:00 / 0:30	1:00 / 0:15
JUMPING JACK	1:00 / 1:00	1:00 / 0:30	1:00 / 0:15
SQUAT	1:00 / 1:00	1:00 / 0:30	1:00 / 0:15
THE MUMMY	1:00 / 1:00	1:00 / 0:30	1:00 / 0:15
SPRINTER SIT-UP	1:00 / 1:00	1:00 / 0:30	1:00 / 0:15
X-JACK	1:00 / 1:00	1:00 / 0:30	1:00 / 0:15
PUSH UP	1:00 / 1:00	1:00 / 0:30	1:00 / 0:15
PIKE	1:00 / 1:00	1:00 / 0:30	1:00 / 0:15
TOTAL TIME	16:00	12:00	10:00

THE CYCLE

TOTAL TIME: 8:00

This workout cycles through a variety of exercises that work your major muscle groups as you move from a standing position to a plank or push-up position and back. The constant change of elevation will drive your heart rate through the roof. Remember: if it doesn't challenge you, it doesn't change you.

For all levels, repeat the set four times. Rest for one minute after each set.

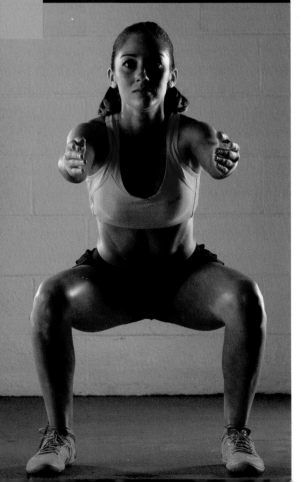

LEVEL 1	WORK	REST
SPRINT	0:20	0:00
SQUAT	0:20	0:00
PLANK HOLD	0:20	0:00

LEVEL 2	WORK	REST
SPRINT	0:20	0:00
SQUAT JUMP	0:20	0:00
BURPEE	0:20	0:00

LEVEL 3	WORK	REST
SPRINT	0:20	0:00
SQUAT PEDAL	0:20	0:00
ALTERNATING LEG LIFT BURPEE	0:20	0:00

CHALLENGE

If you're ready for more, complete all three levels in a "stair step" challenge. Do one set of Level 1, two sets of Level 2, and three sets of Level 3.

BUR-PLEASE!

TOTAL TIME: 7:00

The word "burpee" might elicit a laugh the first time you hear it, but once you've performed one it's far more likely to produce a groan. Loathed by clients and loved by trainers, the burpee is a bastion of the body weight fitness revolution. The explosive movements and changes in elevation raise your heart rate, while the push-up position builds core strength.

Complete as many burpees in each interval as possible, followed by the prescribed period of rest.

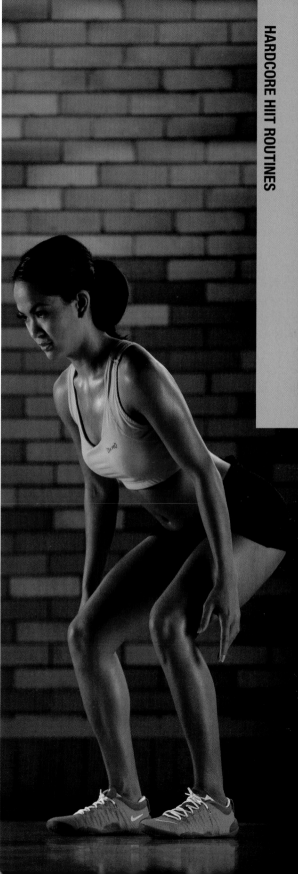

	WORK	REST
BURPEE	0:10	0:10
BURPEE	0:20	0:20
BURPEE	0:20	0:10
BURPEE	0:30	0:30
BURPEE	0:20	0:20
BURPEE	0:30	1:00
BURPEE	0:20	0:20
BURPEE	0:20	0:20
BURPEE	0:10	0:10
BURPEE	0:20	0:20

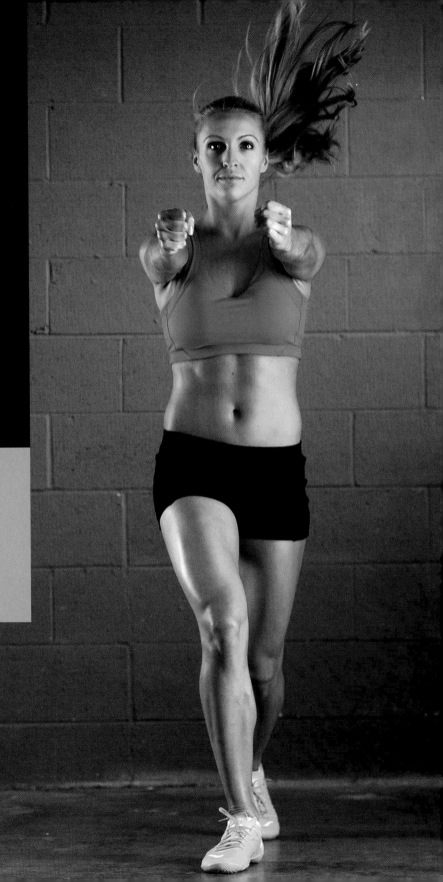

HIIT IT HARD

The heart is the most important muscle in the human body. Like any other muscle, it adapts to the workload it is given. Varying the time, distance, or intensity of your workouts keeps your heart working hard. This longer routine will increase your cardiovascular endurance, improve your athletic performance, and build your strength.

No rest between rounds.

TRAINER TIP

HIIT is a maximal heart rate activity, so you get out what you put in. Push yourself mentally as well as physically with this routine—especially at Level 3. **How much do you want it?**

	LEVEL 1 1 ROUND WORK / REST	LEVEL 2 2 ROUNDS WORK / REST	LEVEL 3 2 ROUNDS WORK / REST
SPRINT	0:30 / 0:30	0:30 / 0:15	0:30 / 0:10
SQUAT	0:30 / 0:30	0:30 / 0:15	0:30 / 0:10
CROSS-COUNTRY SEAL	0:30 / 0:30	0:30 / 0:15	0:30 / 0:10
MOUNTAIN CLIMBER	0:30 / 0:30	0:30 / 0:15	0:30 / 0:10
X-JACK	0:30 / 0:30	0:30 / 0:15	0:30 / 0:10
PUSH-UP JACK	0:30 / 0:30	0:30 / 0:15	0:30 / 0:10
JUMP LUNGE	0:30 / 0:30	0:30 / 0:15	0:30 / 0:10
GRASSHOPPER	0:30 / 0:30	0:30 / 0:15	0:30 / 0:10
TIGER PUSH-UP	0:30 / 0:30	0:30 / 0:15	0:30 / 0:10
BURPEE	0:30 / 0:30	0:30 / 0:15	0:30 / 0:10
TOTAL TIME	10:00	15:00	13:20

FEELING CRABBY?

This routine is named for the crab touch exercise, but HIIT really can help if you're feeling crabby. It decreases inflammation in the brain, improves hormone balance, leads to better mobility, and makes you feel energized and capable. After you blast through this series of exercises, you'll be ready to take on the world.

TRAINER CHALLENGE

Are you up for a challenge? Try the trio! Complete each level three times for nine rounds of increasing difficulty.

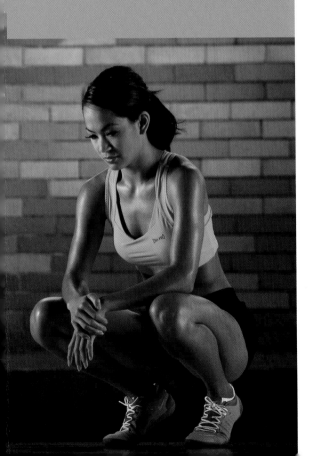

LEVEL 1	WORK	REST
PUSH-UP	0:30	0:00
SQUAT	0:30	0:00
JUMPING JACK	0:30	0:00
PLANK HOLD	0:30	0:00

REPEAT THREE TIMES.
REST FOR ONE MINUTE AFTER EACH SET.
TOTAL TIME: 9:00

LEVEL 2	WORK	REST
CROSS PUSH	0:30	0:00
JUMP LUNGE	0:30	0:00
TRICEP DIP	0:30	0:00
BURPEE	0:30	0:00

REPEAT FIVE TIMES.
REST FOR ONE MINUTE AFTER EACH SET.
TOTAL TIME: 15:00

LEVEL 3	WORK	REST
1-2 PUSH	0:30	0:00
SQUAT PEDAL	0:30	0:00
CRAB TOUCH	0:30	0:00
ALTERNATING LEG LIFT BURPEE	0:30	0:00

REPEAT SEVEN TIMES.
REST FOR ONE MINUTE AFTER EACH SET.
TOTAL TIME: 21:00

OH, MY QUAD

Working big muscles means burning big calories. Banish any thoughts that body weight squats are going to turn you into the Incredible Hulk. The muscles in the lower body—quads, hamstrings, and glutes—are some of the largest in the body and they consume an incredible amount of energy (calories), both while working out and through post exercise "after burn." In addition to making you leaner, squatting improves balance, mobility, and performance, making this a go-to exercise.

SET 1	WORK	REST
SQUAT	0:20	0:00
SQUAT HOLD	0:10	0:00
SQUAT	0:20	0:00
SQUAT HOLD	0:10	0:00
SQUAT	0:20	0:00
SQUAT HOLD	0:10	0:00
SQUAT	0:20	0:00
SQUAT HOLD	0:10	0:00

SET 2	WORK	REST
SQUAT HOLD	0:20	0:00
SQUAT	0:10	0:00
SQUAT HOLD	0:20	0:00
SQUAT	0:10	0:00
SQUAT HOLD	0:20	0:00
SQUAT	0:10	0:00
SQUAT HOLD	0:20	0:00
SQUAT	0:10	0:00

LEVEL 1

DO EACH SET ONCE. REST FOR 1 MINUTE AFTER EACH SET.
TOTAL TIME: 6:00

LEVEL 2

DO EACH SET TWO TIMES. REST FOR ONE MINUTE AFTER EACH SET.
TOTAL TIME: 12:00

LEVEL 3

DO EACH SET THREE TIMES. REST FOR ONE MINUTE AFTER EACH SET.
TOTAL TIME: 18:00

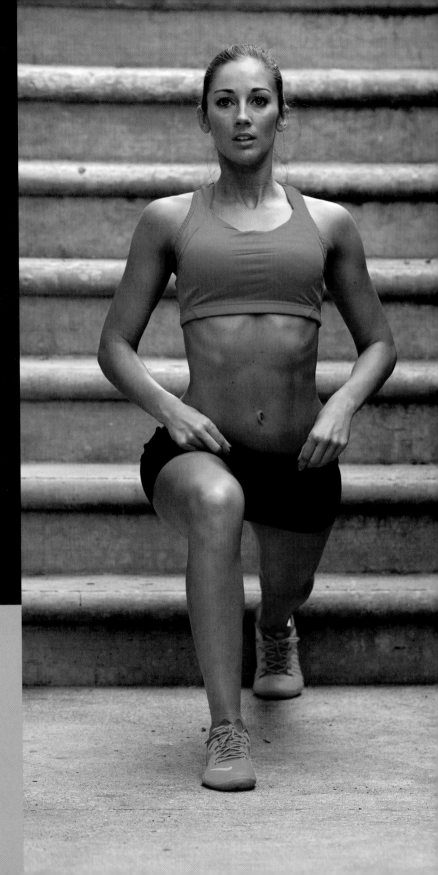

THE TRIFECTA

TOTAL TIME: 7:30

At a 4:1 work-to-rest ratio, this workout will challenge every muscle in your body. Each set is engineered to work as many muscle groups as possible, super-charging your metabolism to incinerate body fat. This is a challenging routine, so form is especially important. Remember that quality trumps quantity. There are no level distinctions on this routine. The goal is to perform as many rounds as you can, with a maximum of three complete rounds.

Rest for 30 seconds after each set.

CAUTION

Pay attention to form on your lunges and squats. Keep your weight in your heels and don't allow your knees to go past your toes.

SET 1	WORK	REST
SPRINT	0:30	0:00
CROSS-COUNTRY SEAL	0:30	0:00
X-JACK	0:30	0:00
MOUNTAIN CLIMBER	0:30	0:00

SET 2	WORK	REST
SQUAT	0:30	0:00
REVERSE LUNGE	0:30	0:00
SQUAT JUMP	0:30	0:00
JUMP LUNGE	0:30	0:00

SET 3	WORK	REST
POWER KNEE (RIGHT)	0:30	0:00
BURPEE	0:30	0:00
POWER KNEE (LEFT)	0:30	0:00
TIGER PUSH-UP	0:30	0:00

JACKED UP

This routine is all jacked up with four very different variations on the classic jumping jack. Each is fun yet challenging, from the cardio-based jacks to the strength-based jacks. The change in pace and elevation, as well as the use of your large muscle groups, will push your heart rate, burn fat, and make you wish those 10-second rests were a little longer. Substitutions are given for the more challenging exercises.

	WORK	REST
JUMPING JACK	0:20	0:10
X-JACK	0:20	0:10
SEAL JACK	0:20	0:10
PUSH-UP JACK	0:20	0:10

LEVEL 1	REPEAT FOUR TIMES. REST FOR 30 SECONDS AFTER EACH SET. **TOTAL TIME: 10:00**
LEVEL 2	REPEAT EIGHT TIMES. REST FOR 30 SECONDS AFTER EACH SET. **TOTAL TIME: 20:00**
LEVEL 3	REPEAT 12 TIMES. REST FOR 30 SECONDS AFTER EACH SET. **TOTAL TIME: 30:00**

TRAINER TIP

For the strength-based jacks, form trumps speed. Keep your chest up and bend from the knees, hips, and ankles for the X-jacks. Make sure your nose touches the floor on the push-up jacks.

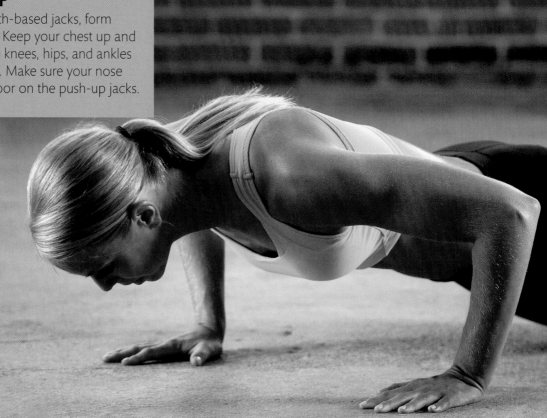

AB-SOLUTELY F-AB-ULOUS!

We all wish for sleek, sexy, defined abs, but abs need to be earned. It will take nutritional discipline and dedication to your training to get the abs you want. The exercises in this routine lift, twist, and turn to activate muscle fibers and get results faster.

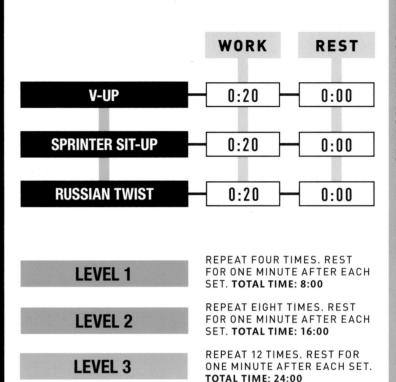

	WORK	REST
V-UP	0:20	0:00
SPRINTER SIT-UP	0:20	0:00
RUSSIAN TWIST	0:20	0:00

LEVEL 1	REPEAT FOUR TIMES. REST FOR ONE MINUTE AFTER EACH SET. **TOTAL TIME: 8:00**
LEVEL 2	REPEAT EIGHT TIMES. REST FOR ONE MINUTE AFTER EACH SET. **TOTAL TIME: 16:00**
LEVEL 3	REPEAT 12 TIMES. REST FOR ONE MINUTE AFTER EACH SET. **TOTAL TIME: 24:00**

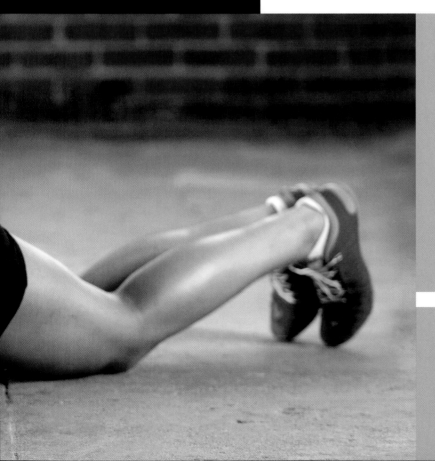

TRAINER TIP

Your core is the area from the bottom of the rib cage to the place where the glutes and hamstring meet. This encompasses the hip flexors, pelvic floor, and glutes. Each of the exercises in this series will require you to engage the core (including hip flexors) and stabilize the spine while moving against your own body weight and gravity.

CHALLENGE

To add additional challenge and resistance to this series, use a medicine ball with each exercise.

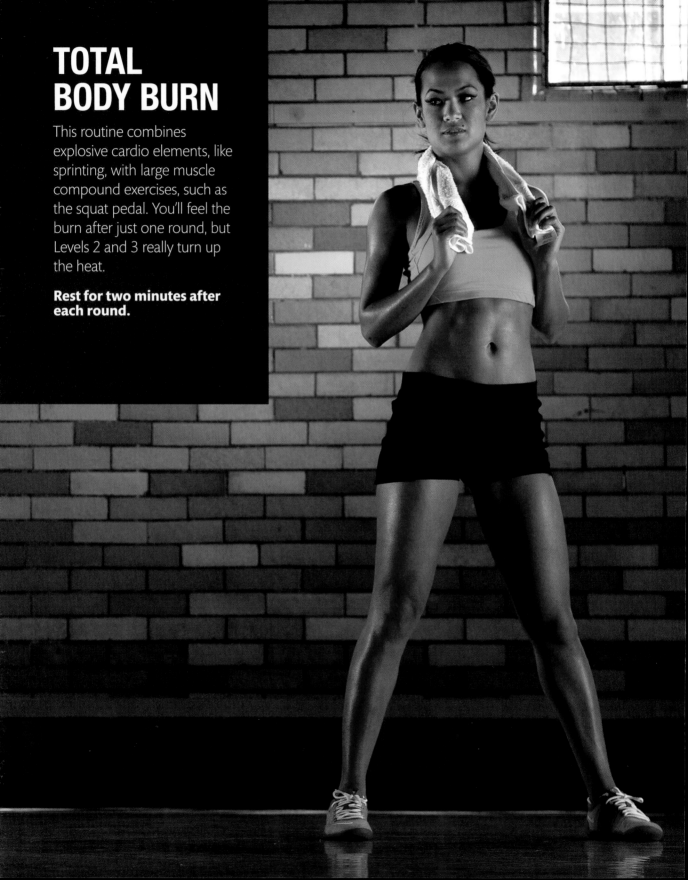

TOTAL BODY BURN

This routine combines explosive cardio elements, like sprinting, with large muscle compound exercises, such as the squat pedal. You'll feel the burn after just one round, but Levels 2 and 3 really turn up the heat.

Rest for two minutes after each round.

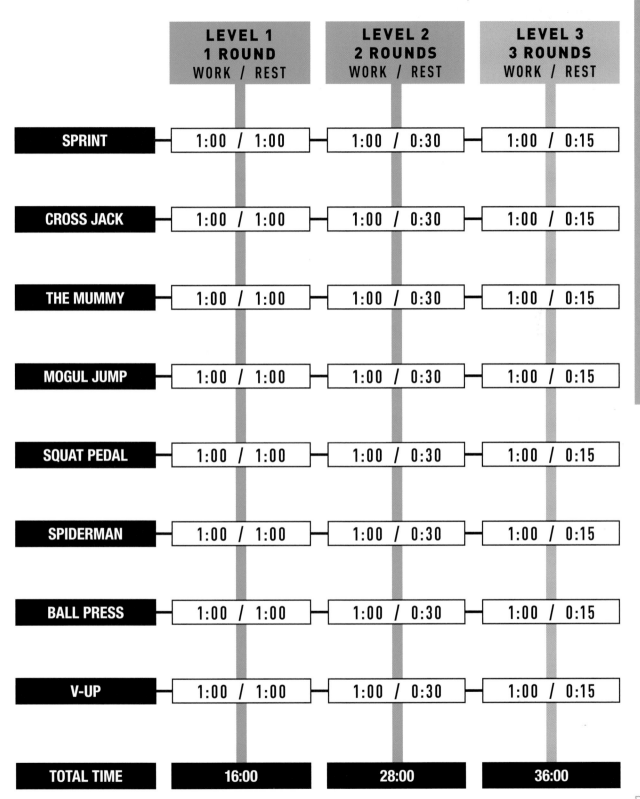

	LEVEL 1 1 ROUND WORK / REST	LEVEL 2 2 ROUNDS WORK / REST	LEVEL 3 3 ROUNDS WORK / REST
SPRINT	1:00 / 1:00	1:00 / 0:30	1:00 / 0:15
CROSS JACK	1:00 / 1:00	1:00 / 0:30	1:00 / 0:15
THE MUMMY	1:00 / 1:00	1:00 / 0:30	1:00 / 0:15
MOGUL JUMP	1:00 / 1:00	1:00 / 0:30	1:00 / 0:15
SQUAT PEDAL	1:00 / 1:00	1:00 / 0:30	1:00 / 0:15
SPIDERMAN	1:00 / 1:00	1:00 / 0:30	1:00 / 0:15
BALL PRESS	1:00 / 1:00	1:00 / 0:30	1:00 / 0:15
V-UP	1:00 / 1:00	1:00 / 0:30	1:00 / 0:15
TOTAL TIME	16:00	28:00	36:00

CORE KILLER

Each exercise in this series will challenge the muscles of the core (six-pack abs, obliques, transverse abs, back, and hips) to work together to stabilize the spine and resist the forces generated by moving your body through space. Unlike doing endless crunches that focus only on the six-pack abs (*rectus abdominis*), these exercises together create a set that will attack your entire core.

CAUTION

Focus on keeping the triangle of your pelvis flat on the floor whenever you are lying on your back. If the curve in your spine becomes exaggerated, you can injure your lower back.

	WORK	REST
V-UP	0:20	0:10
DOUBLE CROSS REACH	0:20	0:10
SPRINTER SIT UP	0:20	0:10
PLANK PUNCH	0:20	0:10

LEVEL 1	REPEAT FOUR TIMES. REST FOR 30 SECONDS AFTER EACH SET. **TOTAL TIME: 10:00**
LEVEL 2	REPEAT SIX TIMES. REST FOR 30 SECONDS AFTER EACH SET. **TOTAL TIME: 15:00**
LEVEL 3	REPEAT EIGHT TIMES. REST FOR 30 SECONDS AFTER EACH SET. **TOTAL TIME: 20:00**

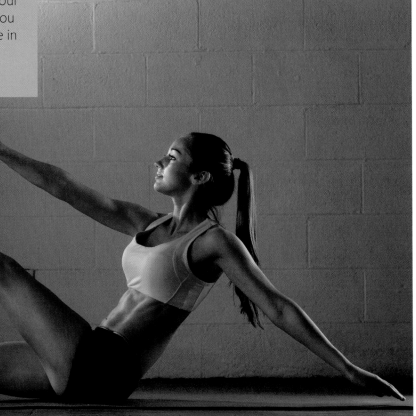

HOP TO HIIT

High energy and high impact, this routine will keep you on your toes. It includes some of my most frequently requested HIIT exercises and will work your entire body: core, legs, glutes, and arms. At a 3:1 work-to-rest ratio, you're going to have to give it all you've got. You can do it!

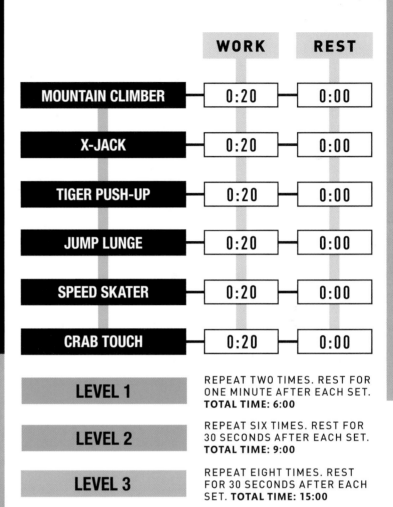

	WORK	REST
MOUNTAIN CLIMBER	0:20	0:00
X-JACK	0:20	0:00
TIGER PUSH-UP	0:20	0:00
JUMP LUNGE	0:20	0:00
SPEED SKATER	0:20	0:00
CRAB TOUCH	0:20	0:00

LEVEL 1	REPEAT TWO TIMES. REST FOR ONE MINUTE AFTER EACH SET. **TOTAL TIME: 6:00**
LEVEL 2	REPEAT SIX TIMES. REST FOR 30 SECONDS AFTER EACH SET. **TOTAL TIME: 9:00**
LEVEL 3	REPEAT EIGHT TIMES. REST FOR 30 SECONDS AFTER EACH SET. **TOTAL TIME: 15:00**

CAUTION

When performing any kind of plyometric (jumping) exercise, the landing and deceleration of the body is incredibly important. Bend softly at the hips, knees, and ankles to control your descent.

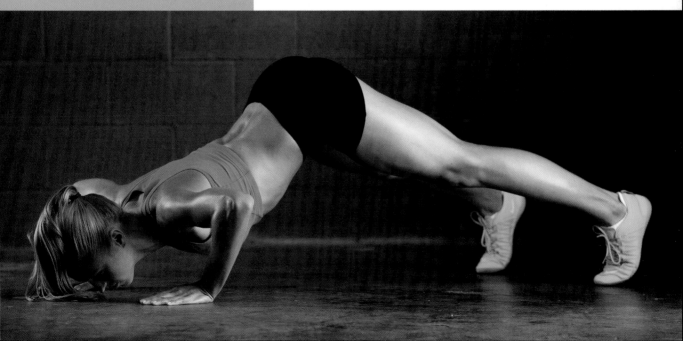

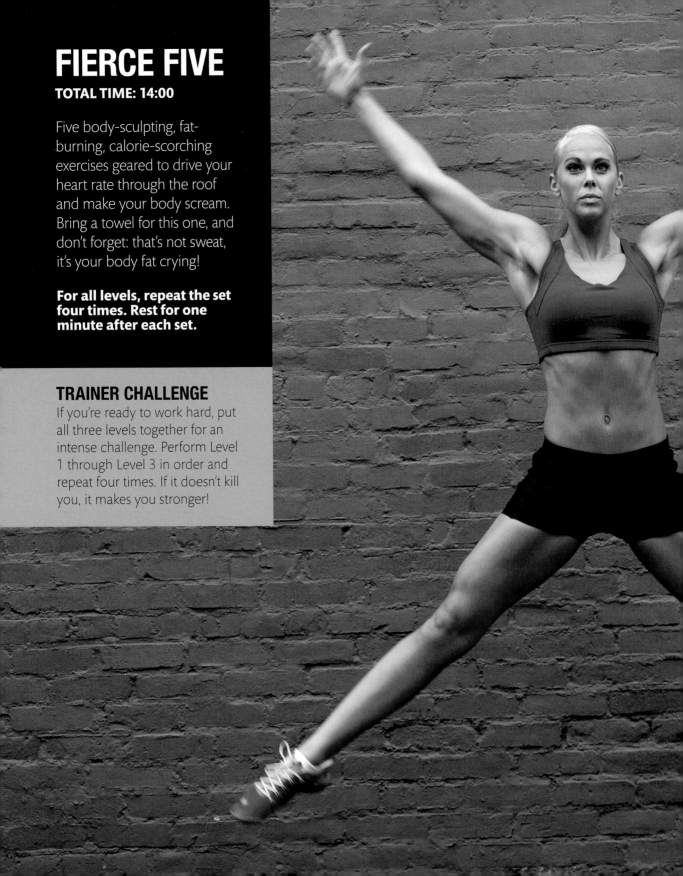

FIERCE FIVE

TOTAL TIME: 14:00

Five body-sculpting, fat-burning, calorie-scorching exercises geared to drive your heart rate through the roof and make your body scream. Bring a towel for this one, and don't forget: that's not sweat, it's your body fat crying!

For all levels, repeat the set four times. Rest for one minute after each set.

TRAINER CHALLENGE

If you're ready to work hard, put all three levels together for an intense challenge. Perform Level 1 through Level 3 in order and repeat four times. If it doesn't kill you, it makes you stronger!

LEVEL 1	WORK	REST
SPRINT	0:30	0:00
PLANK	0:30	0:00
JUMPING JACK	0:30	0:00
PLANK ROTATION	0:30	0:00
SQUAT	0:30	0:00

LEVEL 2	WORK	REST
BURPEE	0:30	0:00
PUSH-UP	0:30	0:00
SEAL JACK	0:30	0:00
PLANK PUNCH	0:30	0:00
SQUAT JUMP	0:30	0:00

LEVEL 3	WORK	REST
ALTERNATING LEG LIFT BURPEE	0:30	0:00
1-2 PUSH	0:30	0:00
STAR	0:30	0:00
IN-AND-OUT ABS	0:30	0:00
SQUAT PEDAL	0:30	0:00

"T" IT UP

Single leg exercises engage smaller muscles like the abductors, *gluteus medius*, and *quadratus lumborum* in ways that can't be replicated with both feet on the floor. When you remove the support of one leg, your coordination, balance, and stabilization are all challenged, which leads to huge performance gains, particularly if you are an athlete.

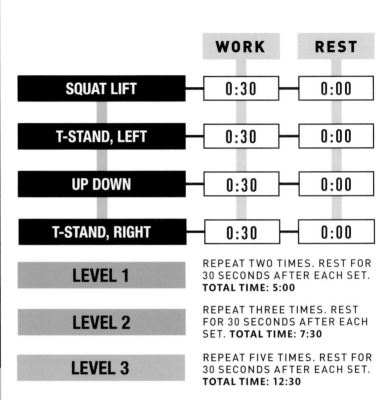

	WORK	REST
SQUAT LIFT	0:30	0:00
T-STAND, LEFT	0:30	0:00
UP DOWN	0:30	0:00
T-STAND, RIGHT	0:30	0:00
LEVEL 1	REPEAT TWO TIMES. REST FOR 30 SECONDS AFTER EACH SET. **TOTAL TIME: 5:00**	
LEVEL 2	REPEAT THREE TIMES. REST FOR 30 SECONDS AFTER EACH SET. **TOTAL TIME: 7:30**	
LEVEL 3	REPEAT FIVE TIMES. REST FOR 30 SECONDS AFTER EACH SET. **TOTAL TIME: 12:30**	

CHALLENGE

To increase the challenge and calorie burn of these exercises, try incorporating a weight (medicine ball, dumbbell, or kettlebell). Do not add the weight until you are confident using only your body weight as resistance.

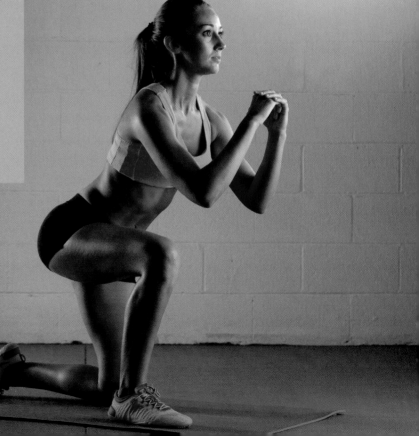

HARD-CORE

The core muscles work as stabilizers for the entire body and help the body function more effectively. Core muscles like the *rectus abdominis* (six-pack abs), the internal and external obliques, the *transverse abdominis*, and the *erector spinae* work together to supply strength and coordinated movement.

	WORK	REST
BICYCLE CRUNCH	0:30	0:00
SIDE PLANK, RIGHT	0:30	0:00
RUSSIAN TWIST	0:30	0:00
SIDE PLANK, LEFT	0:30	0:00

LEVEL 1	REPEAT TWO TIMES. REST FOR 30 SECONDS AFTER EACH SET. TOTAL TIME: 5:00
LEVEL 2	REPEAT THREE TIMES. REST FOR 30 SECONDS AFTER EACH SET. TOTAL TIME: 7:30
LEVEL 3	REPEAT FIVE TIMES. REST FOR 30 SECONDS AFTER EACH SET. TOTAL TIME: 12:30

TRAINER TIP

There are many benefits to strengthening your core, including improved functional fitness, correct posture, a toned tummy, injury prevention, and increased athletic performance. However, the muscles that comprise your core need rest and recovery. Try to avoid back-to-back workouts that isolate your core muscles.

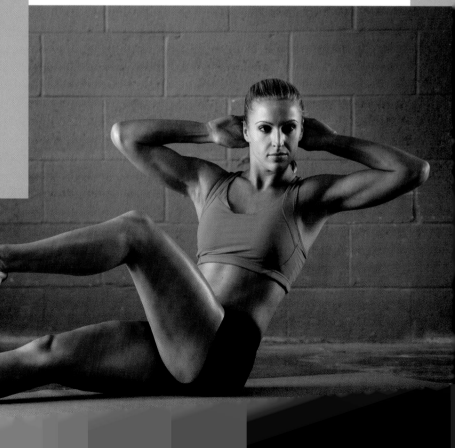

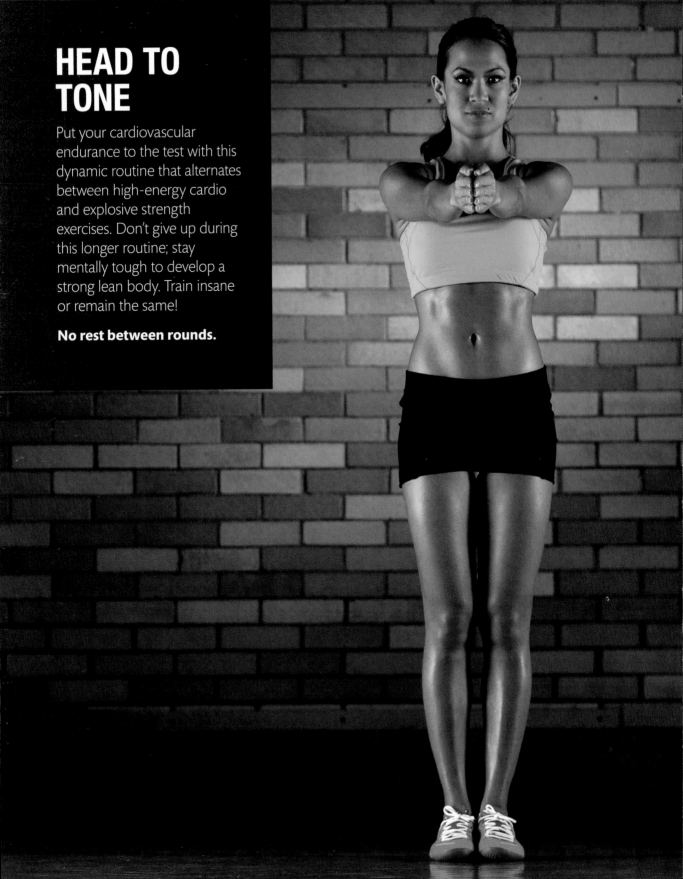

HEAD TO TONE

Put your cardiovascular endurance to the test with this dynamic routine that alternates between high-energy cardio and explosive strength exercises. Don't give up during this longer routine; stay mentally tough to develop a strong lean body. Train insane or remain the same!

No rest between rounds.

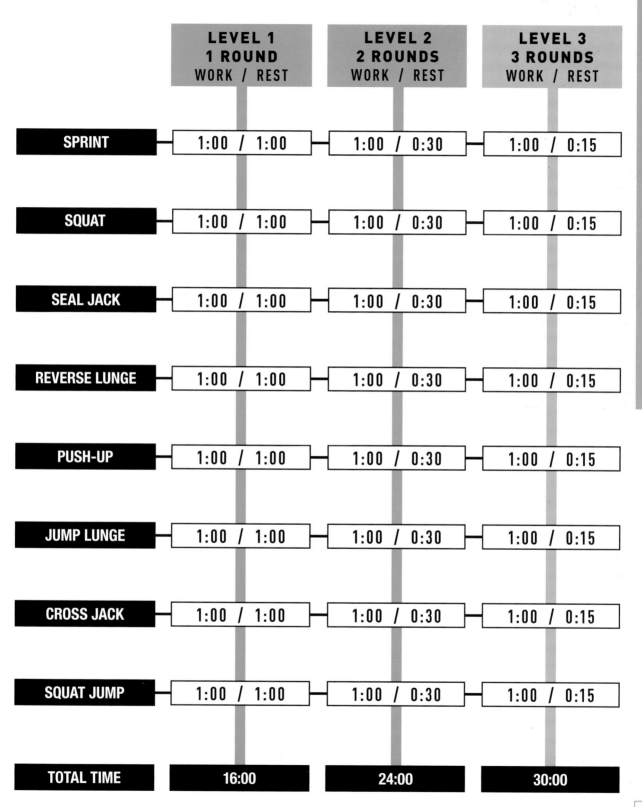

	LEVEL 1 **1 ROUND** WORK / REST	**LEVEL 2** **2 ROUNDS** WORK / REST	**LEVEL 3** **3 ROUNDS** WORK / REST
SPRINT	1:00 / 1:00	1:00 / 0:30	1:00 / 0:15
SQUAT	1:00 / 1:00	1:00 / 0:30	1:00 / 0:15
SEAL JACK	1:00 / 1:00	1:00 / 0:30	1:00 / 0:15
REVERSE LUNGE	1:00 / 1:00	1:00 / 0:30	1:00 / 0:15
PUSH-UP	1:00 / 1:00	1:00 / 0:30	1:00 / 0:15
JUMP LUNGE	1:00 / 1:00	1:00 / 0:30	1:00 / 0:15
CROSS JACK	1:00 / 1:00	1:00 / 0:30	1:00 / 0:15
SQUAT JUMP	1:00 / 1:00	1:00 / 0:30	1:00 / 0:15
TOTAL TIME	16:00	24:00	30:00

STAR POWER

Yelling, "I'm a star!" as loudly as possible is optional during this routine, but highly recommended. That brief moment of levity may make you forget how much your legs and lungs are burning during this blockbuster workout.

CAUTION

When performing X-jacks and stars, it's easy to overcompensate by bending from the hips when landing. If you're looking at the floor, there's a good chance this is happening. In time it will stress your lower back, so keep your chest up, look forward, and engage your core.

	WORK	REST
X-JACK	0:20	0:10
JUMP LUNGE	0:20	0:10
STAR	0:20	0:10
CROSS PUSH	0:20	0:10

LEVEL 1 — REPEAT TWO TIMES. REST FOR 30 SECONDS AFTER EACH SET. **TOTAL TIME: 5:00**

LEVEL 2 — REPEAT FOUR TIMES. REST FOR 30 SECONDS AFTER EACH SET. **TOTAL TIME: 10:00**

LEVEL 3 — REPEAT SIX TIMES. REST FOR 30 SECONDS AFTER EACH SET. **TOTAL TIME: 15:00**

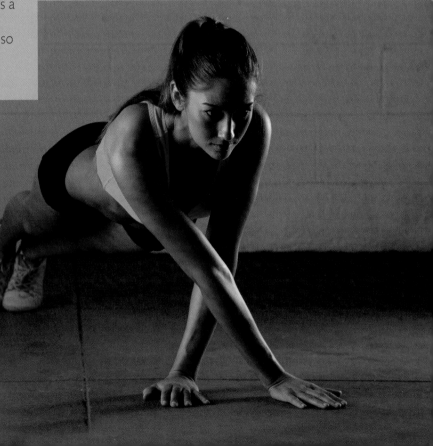

SPRINT FOR HIIT

Sprinting is arguably one of the most challenging forms of exercise. It requires you to run as hard as you possibly can, focusing all your energy and power into short, intense bursts. The benefits of sprinting are worth the effort, as it raises your anaerobic threshold and obliterates calories in the process.

TRAINER TIP

When sprinting, relax your hands and shoulders, keep your torso tall, and engage your core. Drive with your arms to create momentum but keep the arms bent at roughly 90 degrees and swing your hands from shoulders to buttocks.

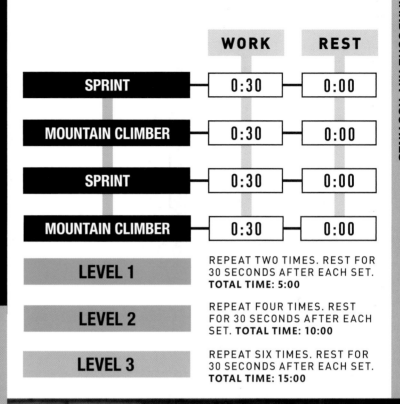

	WORK	REST
SPRINT	0:30	0:00
MOUNTAIN CLIMBER	0:30	0:00
SPRINT	0:30	0:00
MOUNTAIN CLIMBER	0:30	0:00
LEVEL 1	REPEAT TWO TIMES. REST FOR 30 SECONDS AFTER EACH SET. **TOTAL TIME: 5:00**	
LEVEL 2	REPEAT FOUR TIMES. REST FOR 30 SECONDS AFTER EACH SET. **TOTAL TIME: 10:00**	
LEVEL 3	REPEAT SIX TIMES. REST FOR 30 SECONDS AFTER EACH SET. **TOTAL TIME: 15:00**	

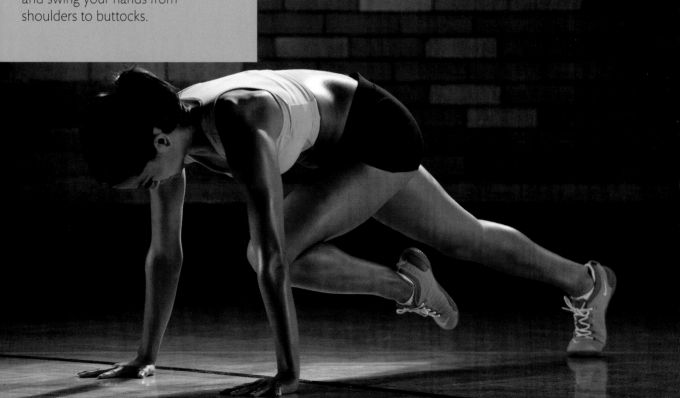

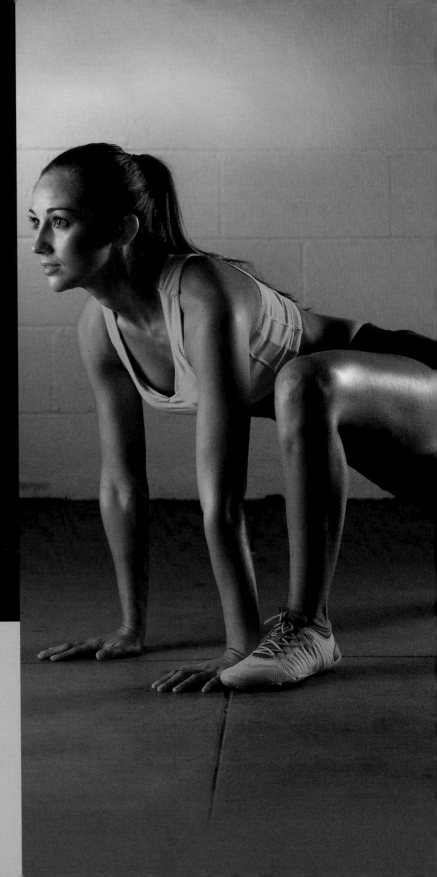

THE TERRIBLE TRIO

TOTAL TIME: 18:00

You'll discover that three really is the magic number in this total body challenge: 3 exercises × 3 sets × 3 rounds. Each set blends high-output cardio with leg-shaking, arm-quivering strength exercises. You're going to have to dig deep and push for this one.

Repeat each set three times before moving to the next set. Rest 30 seconds at the end of each round.

CHALLENGE

Test your cardiovascular endurance by removing the rest between sets. Complete each set in order (nine exercises), then rest for one minute and repeat twice more for a total of three full rounds. Good luck!

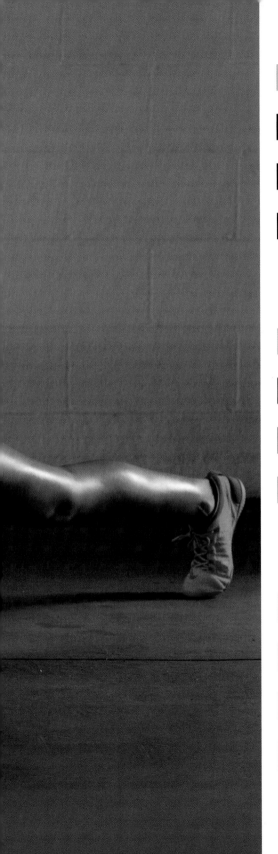

SET 1 (3 ROUNDS)	WORK	REST
CROSS-COUNTRY SEAL	0:30	0:00
JUMP LUNGE	0:30	0:00
MOUNTAIN CLIMBER	0:30	0:00

SET 2 (3 ROUNDS)	WORK	REST
SPRINT	0:30	0:00
1-2 PUSH	0:30	0:00
BURPEE	0:30	0:00

SET 3 (3 ROUNDS)	WORK	REST
STAR	0:30	0:00
SQUAT PEDAL	0:30	0:00
GRASSHOPPER	0:30	0:00

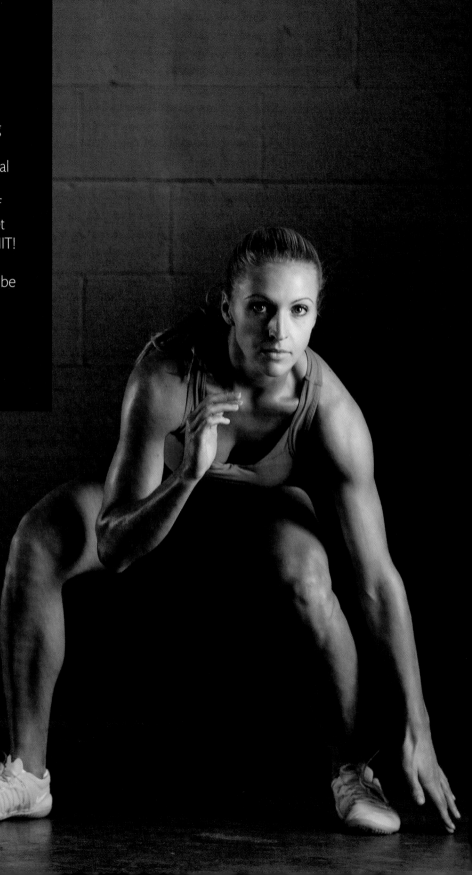

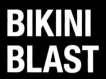

BIKINI
BLAST

After five years of preparing the Indianapolis Colts Cheerleaders for their annual swimsuit calendar I have earned the unofficial title of "Bikini Whisperer." My secret weapon—lots and lots of HIIT! Follow this fast-paced total body workout and you will be bikini ready in no time.

Rest for one minute after each round.

	LEVEL 1 1 ROUND WORK / REST	LEVEL 2 2 ROUNDS WORK / REST	LEVEL 3 3 ROUNDS WORK / REST
SPRINT	0:30 / 0:30	0:30 / 0:15	0:30 / 0:10
MOUNTAIN CLIMBER	0:30 / 0:30	0:30 / 0:15	0:30 / 0:10
CROSS JACK	0:30 / 0:30	0:30 / 0:15	0:30 / 0:10
CRAB TOUCH	0:30 / 0:30	0:30 / 0:15	0:30 / 0:10
SIDE SUICIDES	0:30 / 0:30	0:30 / 0:15	0:30 / 0:10
TIGER PUSH-UP	0:30 / 0:30	0:30 / 0:15	0:30 / 0:10
SKATER JUMP	0:30 / 0:30	0:30 / 0:15	0:30 / 0:10
RUSSIAN TWIST	0:30 / 0:30	0:30 / 0:15	0:30 / 0:10
TOTAL TIME	8:00	14:00	19:00

DROP IT LIKE IT'S SQUAT

Squats trigger all of the large muscles in the lower body, particularly the quads, hamstrings, and glutes. They also require core stabilization and hip and ankle mobility, making the squat a perfect exercise to attain your workout goals.

CAUTION

Proper form is critical when performing squats, but it's easy to get lazy, especially when doing a lot at once. Don't drop your chest, don't allow your knees to buckle inward, and keep your knees behind your toes.

	WORK	REST
SQUAT	0:20	0:10
LATERAL LUNGE, RIGHT	0:20	0:10
SQUAT HOLD	0:20	0:10
LATERAL LUNGE, LEFT	0:20	0:10
SQUAT HOLD	0:20	0:10
SQUAT LIFT, RIGHT	0:20	0:10
SQUAT HOLD	0:20	0:10
SQUAT LIFT, LEFT	0:20	0:10

LEVEL 1	DO ONE SET. **TOTAL TIME: 4:00**
LEVEL 2	DO TWO SETS. REST FOR 30 SECONDS AFTER EACH SET. **TOTAL TIME: 9:00**
LEVEL 3	DO THREE SETS. REST FOR 30 SECONDS AFTER EACH SET. **TOTAL TIME: 13:30**

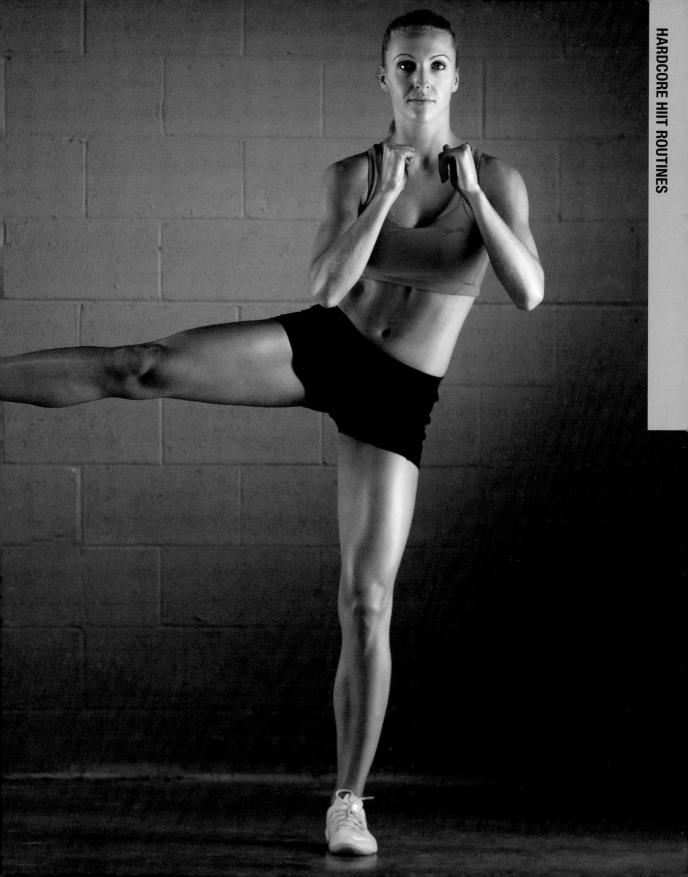

ROW NO YOU DON'T!

Rowing is great cardiovascular exercise that requires equal effort from your upper and lower body, building muscular endurance and core strength. This routine couples row boats with two other core-focused total body exercises. All three exercises activate both upper and lower body simultaneously while engaging the abs and back for stability and strength.

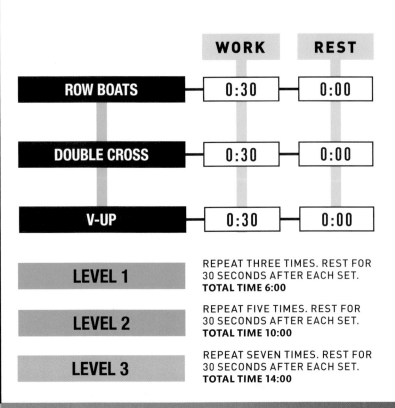

	WORK	REST
ROW BOATS	0:30	0:00
DOUBLE CROSS	0:30	0:00
V-UP	0:30	0:00

LEVEL 1	REPEAT THREE TIMES. REST FOR 30 SECONDS AFTER EACH SET. **TOTAL TIME 6:00**
LEVEL 2	REPEAT FIVE TIMES. REST FOR 30 SECONDS AFTER EACH SET. **TOTAL TIME 10:00**
LEVEL 3	REPEAT SEVEN TIMES. REST FOR 30 SECONDS AFTER EACH SET. **TOTAL TIME 14:00**

CHALLENGE
Incorporating a weight (medicine ball, dumbell, or kettlebell) with these exercises will increase the challenge and the calorie burn. However, do not add the weight until you are confident and stable using only your body weight as resistance.

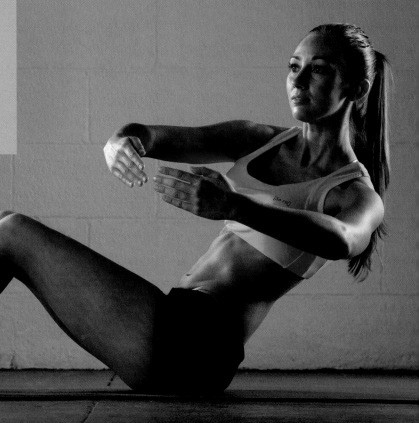

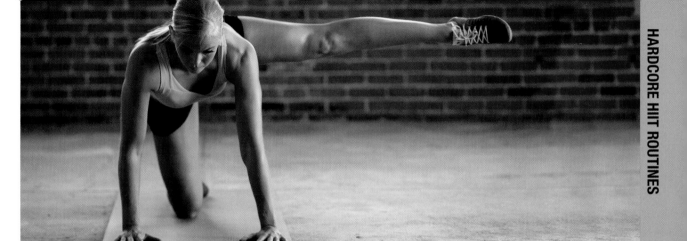

BUTT BUSTERS

TOTAL TIME: 18:00

Build a bulletproof butt with this routine! The large and small muscles of the butt, hips, and legs are activated simultaneously, giving you the toned, tight, and round derrière of your dreams.

Do each set three times. Rest for 30 seconds after each set.

SET 1	WORK	REST
SQUAT	0:30	0:00
ROTATED DONKEY KICK (RIGHT)	0:30	0:00
LATERAL SWEEP (LEFT)	0:30	0:00

SET 2	WORK	REST
REVERSE LUNGE	0:30	0:00
ROTATED DONKEY KICK (LEFT)	0:30	0:00
LATERAL SWEEP (LEFT)	0:30	0:00

SET 3	WORK	REST
IN AND OUTS	0:30	0:00
LATERAL LUNGE	0:30	0:00
SQUAT PEDAL	0:30	0:00

IT'S NOT EASY BEING LEAN

This metabolic-boosting routine is designed to push your limits. Give it all you have and work at maximal heart rate to extend the "after burn" effect of HIIT well beyond the time it takes to complete this head-to-toe total body workout.

CHALLENGE

If you're up for a challenge, test your cardiovascular endurance by removing the rest between sets. Complete each set in order (12 exercises), then rest for one minute. Do this three times. Good Luck!

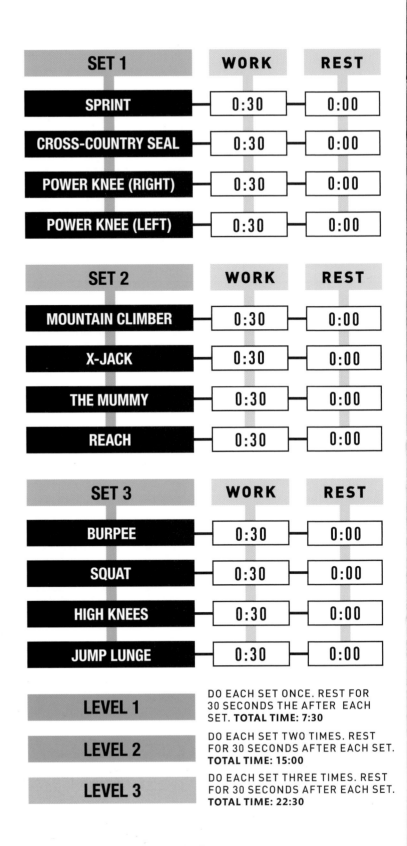

SET 1	WORK	REST
SPRINT	0:30	0:00
CROSS-COUNTRY SEAL	0:30	0:00
POWER KNEE (RIGHT)	0:30	0:00
POWER KNEE (LEFT)	0:30	0:00

SET 2	WORK	REST
MOUNTAIN CLIMBER	0:30	0:00
X-JACK	0:30	0:00
THE MUMMY	0:30	0:00
REACH	0:30	0:00

SET 3	WORK	REST
BURPEE	0:30	0:00
SQUAT	0:30	0:00
HIGH KNEES	0:30	0:00
JUMP LUNGE	0:30	0:00

LEVEL 1	DO EACH SET ONCE. REST FOR 30 SECONDS THE AFTER EACH SET. **TOTAL TIME: 7:30**
LEVEL 2	DO EACH SET TWO TIMES. REST FOR 30 SECONDS AFTER EACH SET. **TOTAL TIME: 15:00**
LEVEL 3	DO EACH SET THREE TIMES. REST FOR 30 SECONDS AFTER EACH SET. **TOTAL TIME: 22:30**

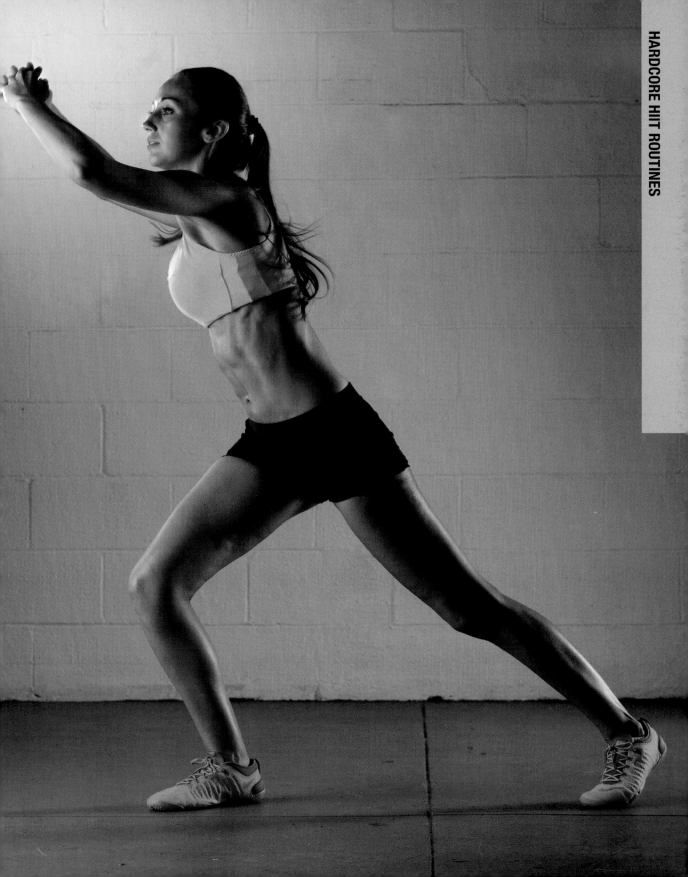

FIRM AND BURN

Who doesn't want to firm and burn? This series of short 4:1 work-to-rest ratio intervals will require maximum effort for maximum effect.

TRAINER CHALLENGE

For an intense 45-minute challenge, perform three rounds of each level. Start with Level 1 and finish with Level 3.

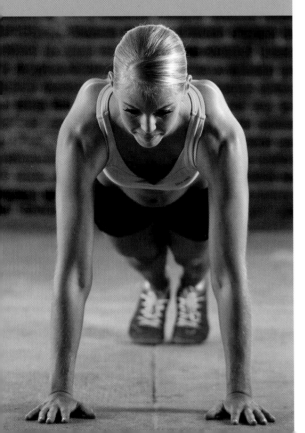

LEVEL 1	WORK	REST
JUMPING JACK	0:30	0:00
CROSS-COUNTRY SEAL	0:30	0:00
X-JACK	0:30	0:00
MOUNTAIN CLIMBER	0:30	0:00

REPEAT THREE TIMES.
REST FOR 30 SECONDS AFTER EACH SET.
TOTAL TIME: 7:30

LEVEL 2

SET 1	WORK	REST
MOUNTAIN CLIMBER	0:30	0:00
THE MUMMY	0:30	0:00
PUSH-UP	0:30	0:00
SEAL JACK	0:30	0:00

SET 2	WORK	REST
SQUAT	0:30	0:00
SQUAT HOLD	0:30	0:00
SQUAT	0:30	0:00
SQUAT HOLD	0:30	0:00

REPEAT THREE TIMES.
REST FOR 30 SECONDS AFTER EACH SET.
TOTAL TIME: 15:00

LEVEL 3

SET 1	WORK	REST
SPRINT	0:30	0:00
1-2 PUSH	0:30	0:00
CRAB TOUCH	0:30	0:00
SQUAT JUMP	0:30	0:00

SET 2	WORK	REST
PEDAL	0:30	0:00
SQUAT LIFT (RIGHT)	0:30	0:00
SKI SQUAT	0:30	0:00
SQUAT LIFT (LEFT)	0:30	0:00

SET 3	WORK	REST
CROSS PUSH	0:30	0:00
4 CALF RAISES + 4 TAPS	0:30	0:00
REACH	0:30	0:00
UP DOWN	0:30	0:00

REPEAT THREE TIMES.
REST FOR 30 SECONDS AFTER EACH SET.
TOTAL TIME: 22:30

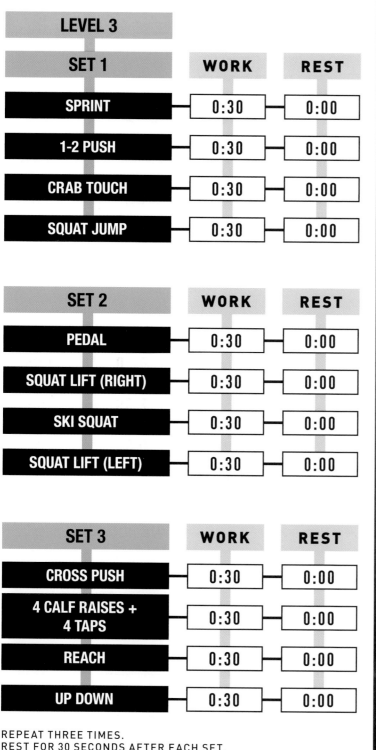

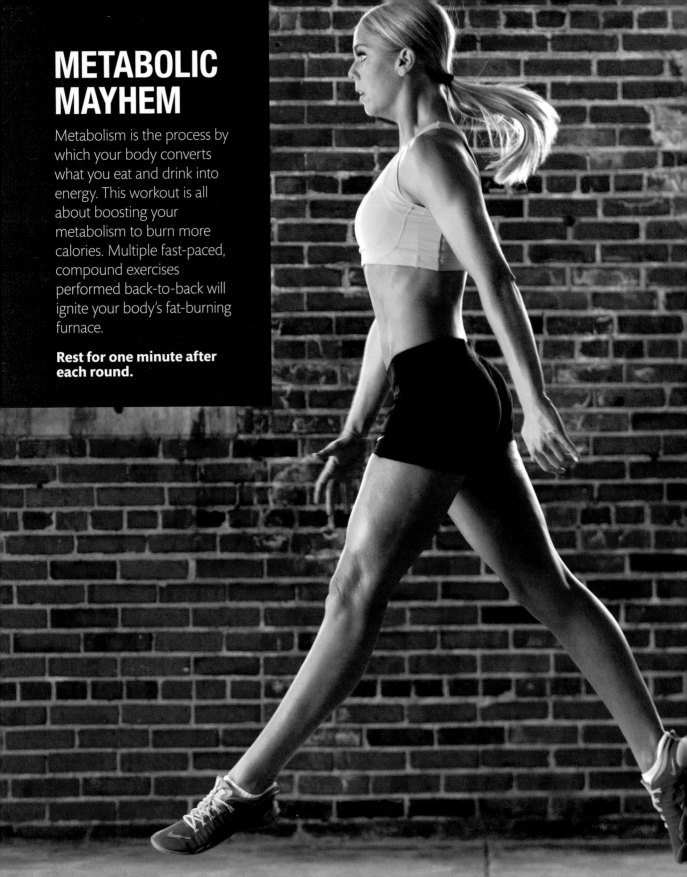

METABOLIC MAYHEM

Metabolism is the process by which your body converts what you eat and drink into energy. This workout is all about boosting your metabolism to burn more calories. Multiple fast-paced, compound exercises performed back-to-back will ignite your body's fat-burning furnace.

Rest for one minute after each round.

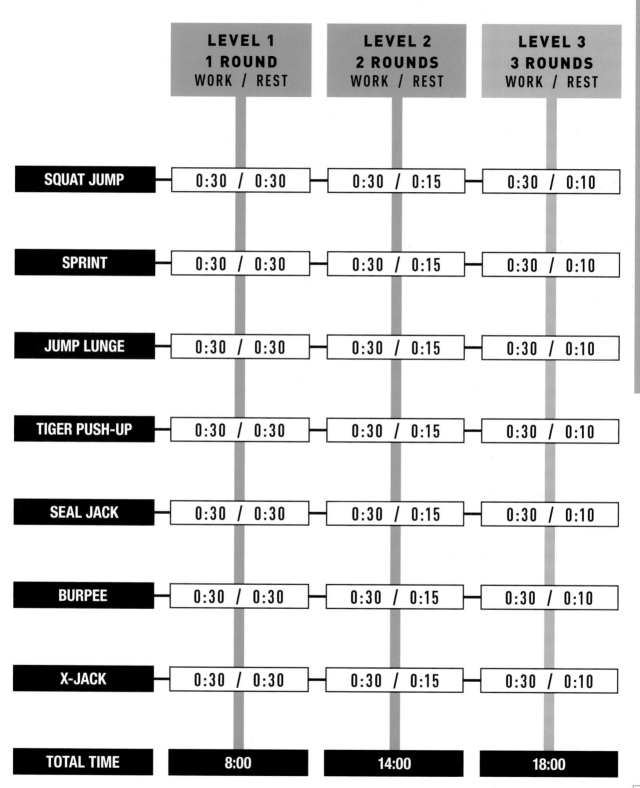

	LEVEL 1 1 ROUND WORK / REST	LEVEL 2 2 ROUNDS WORK / REST	LEVEL 3 3 ROUNDS WORK / REST
SQUAT JUMP	0:30 / 0:30	0:30 / 0:15	0:30 / 0:10
SPRINT	0:30 / 0:30	0:30 / 0:15	0:30 / 0:10
JUMP LUNGE	0:30 / 0:30	0:30 / 0:15	0:30 / 0:10
TIGER PUSH-UP	0:30 / 0:30	0:30 / 0:15	0:30 / 0:10
SEAL JACK	0:30 / 0:30	0:30 / 0:15	0:30 / 0:10
BURPEE	0:30 / 0:30	0:30 / 0:15	0:30 / 0:10
X-JACK	0:30 / 0:30	0:30 / 0:15	0:30 / 0:10
TOTAL TIME	8:00	14:00	18:00

4 IN 4

TOTAL TIME: 4:00

Short on time or looking for a metabolic boost? I have you covered with these four-minute "finishers." Each short, total-body routine will spike your heart rate and kick your metabolism into gear for that post-HIIT after burn.

Perform these routines as a stand-alone workout if pressed for time, or add them to the end of a resistance-training workout as a calorie scorching finish. No rest between rounds!

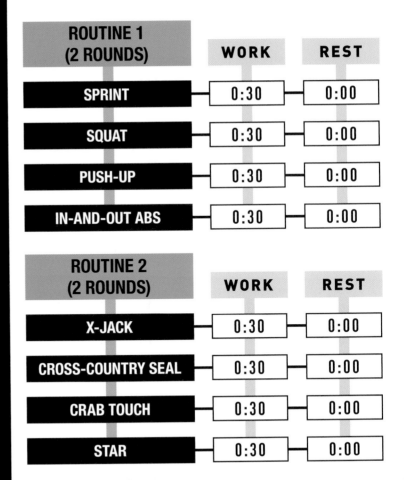

ROUTINE 1 (2 ROUNDS)	WORK	REST
SPRINT	0:30	0:00
SQUAT	0:30	0:00
PUSH-UP	0:30	0:00
IN-AND-OUT ABS	0:30	0:00

ROUTINE 2 (2 ROUNDS)	WORK	REST
X-JACK	0:30	0:00
CROSS-COUNTRY SEAL	0:30	0:00
CRAB TOUCH	0:30	0:00
STAR	0:30	0:00

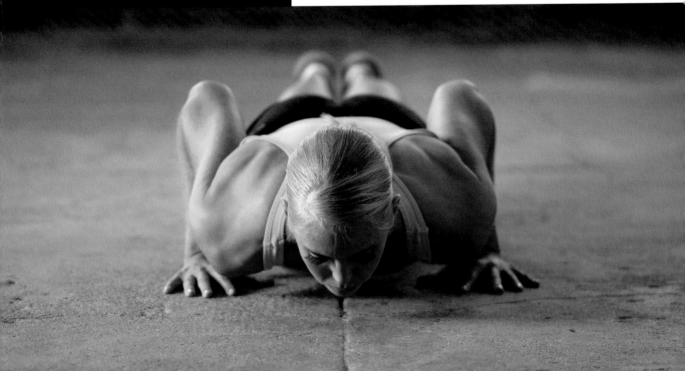

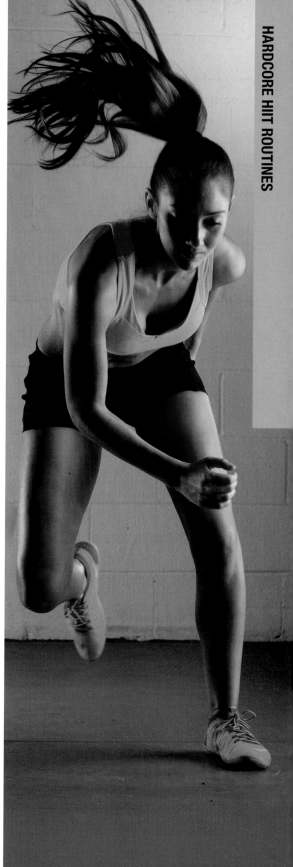

ROUTINE 3 (1 ROUND)	WORK	REST
SPRINT	0:30	0:00
SPIDERMAN	0:30	0:00
UP DOWN	0:30	0:00
1-2 PUSH	0:30	0:00
POWER KNEE (RIGHT)	0:30	0:00
SQUAT JUMP	0:30	0:00
POWER KNEE (LEFT)	0:30	0:00
BURPEE	0:30	0:00

ROUTINE 4 (1 ROUND)	WORK	REST
BURPEE	0:30	0:00
JUMP LUNGE	0:30	0:00
CROSS PUSH	0:30	0:00
CROSS JACK	0:30	0:00
SQUAT PEDAL	0:30	0:00
TIGER PUSH-UP	0:30	0:00
MOGUL JUMP	0:30	0:00
V-UP	0:30	0:00

PERFECT TENS

TOTAL TIME: 10:00

Four radically different 10-minute routines geared to make you sweat, torch calories, and give you that workout buzz you crave. These routines may be short, but that doesn't mean they're easy. Choose the level that's right for you, work hard, and push yourself!

TOP TEN

LEVEL 1

REPEAT TWO TIMES.

	WORK	REST
SPRINT	0:20	0:10
SQUAT	0:20	0:10
CROSS JACK	0:20	0:10
REVERSE LUNGE	0:20	0:10
SEAL JACK	0:20	0:10
PUSH-UP	0:20	0:10
THE MUMMY	0:20	0:10
4 CALF RAISES + 4 TAPS	0:20	0:10
TRICEP DIP	0:20	0:10
BICYCLE CRUNCH	0:20	0:10

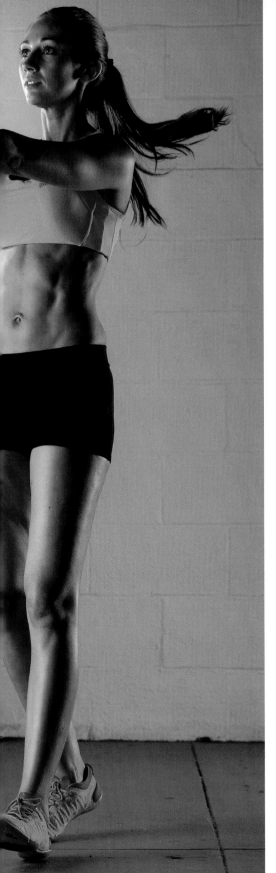

CARDIO ABS

LEVEL 2

SET 1 (3 ROUNDS)	WORK	REST
MOUNTAIN CLIMBER	0:30	0:00
ROW BOAT	0:30	0:00
BICYCLE CRUNCH	0:30	0:00
V-UP	0:30	0:00

SET 2 (2 ROUNDS)	REST FOR 30 SECONDS BETWEEN ROUNDS.	
BURPEE	0:20	0:10
1-2 PUSH	0:20	0:10
GRASSHOPPER	0:20	0:10
PLANK PUNCH	0:20	0:10

THE COMPLETE REPEAT

LEVEL 2 OR LEVEL 3

SET 1 (3 ROUNDS)	WORK	REST
SPRINT	0:30	0:00
X-JACK	0:30	0:00
CROSS-COUNTRY SEAL	0:30	0:00
HIGH KNEES	0:30	0:00

SET 2 (2 ROUNDS)	REST FOR 30 SECONDS BETWEEN ROUNDS.	
SQUAT JUMP	0:20	0:10
TIGER PUSH-UP	0:20	0:10
JUMP LUNGE	0:20	0:10
SPHINX	0:20	0:10

SHOTGUN SETS

LEVEL 3	ROUND 1		ROUND 2	
DO EACH ROUND ONE TIME. REST FOR ONE MINUTE BETWEEN ROUNDS.	WORK	REST	WORK	REST
SPRINT	0:20	0:10	0:20	0:10
SQUAT	0:20	0:10	0:20	0:10
CROSS-COUNTRY SEAL	0:20	0:10	0:20	0:10
PUSH-UP	0:20	0:10	0:20	0:10
CROSS JACK	0:20	0:10	0:20	0:10
REVERSE LUNGE	0:20	0:10	0:20	0:10
BURPEE	0:20	0:10	0:20	0:10
TRICEP DIP	0:20	0:10	0:20	0:10
STAR	0:20	0:10	0:20	0:10
CRAB TOUCH	0:20	0:10	0:20	0:10
THE MUMMY	0:20	0:10	0:20	0:10
BALL PRESS	0:20	0:10	0:20	0:10
POWER KNEE (RIGHT)	0:20	0:10	0:20	0:10
SQUAT LIFT (RIGHT)	0:20	0:10	0:20	0:10
POWER KNEE (LEFT)	0:20	0:10	0:20	0:10
SQUAT LIFT (LEFT)	0:20	0:10	0:20	0:10
SIDE SUICIDES	0:20	0:10	0:20	0:10
CROSS PUSH	0:20	0:10	0:20	0:10

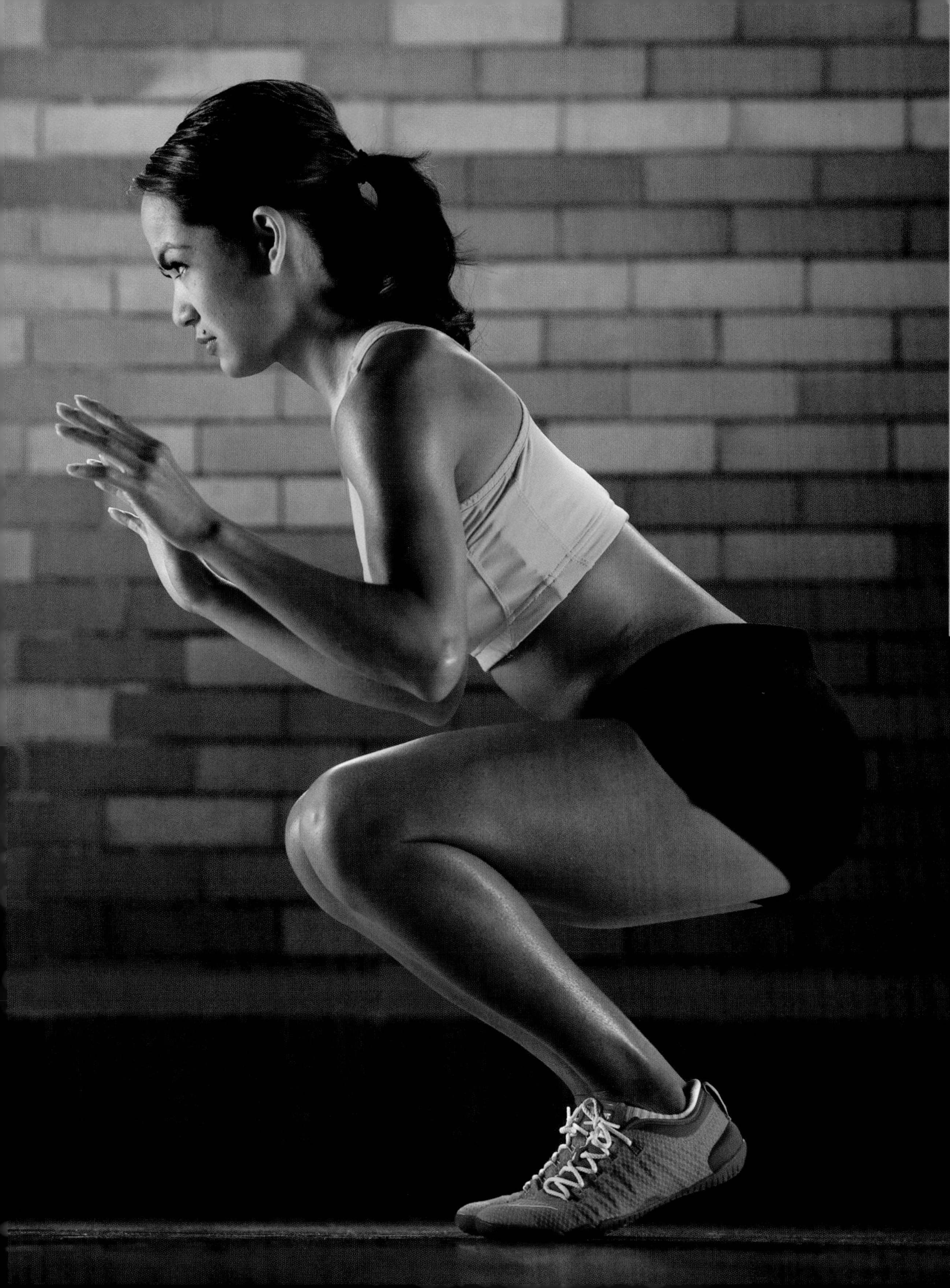

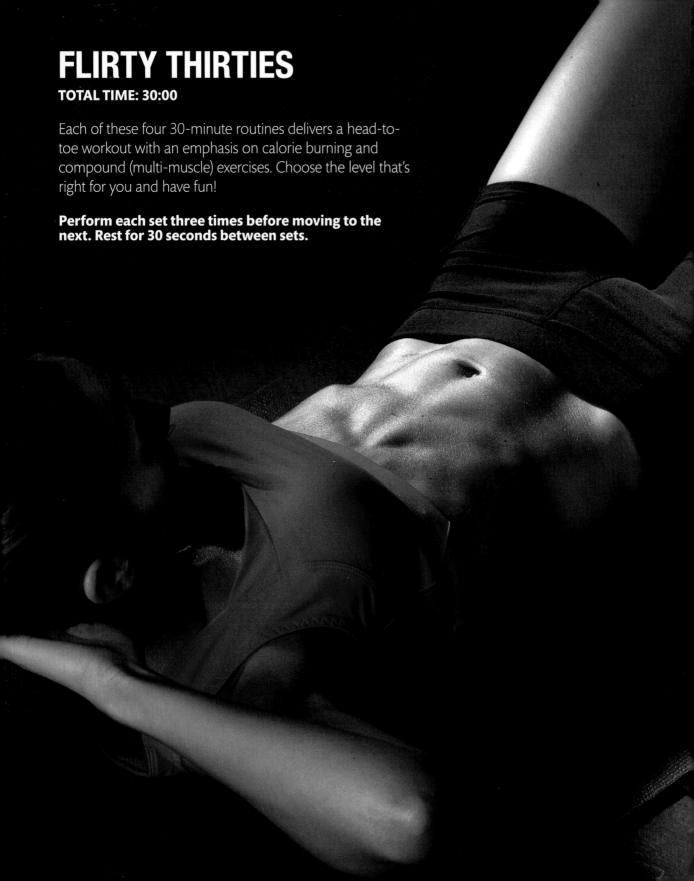

FLIRTY THIRTIES

TOTAL TIME: 30:00

Each of these four 30-minute routines delivers a head-to-toe workout with an emphasis on calorie burning and compound (multi-muscle) exercises. Choose the level that's right for you and have fun!

Perform each set three times before moving to the next. Rest for 30 seconds between sets.

TOTAL TONER

LEVEL 1 OR LEVEL 2

SET 1 (3 ROUNDS)	WORK
SPRINT	0:30
HIGH KNEES	0:30
JUMPING JACK	0:30
THE MUMMY	0:30

SET 2 (3 ROUNDS)	WORK
SQUAT	0:30
REVERSE LUNGE	0:30
LATERAL LUNGE	0:30
SQUAT HOLD	0:30

SET 3 (3 ROUNDS)	WORK
PLANK	0:30
CROSS JACK	0:30
PUSH-UP	0:30
TRICEP DIP	0:30

SET 4 (3 ROUNDS)	WORK
PIKE	0:30
SIDE BEND (RIGHT)	0:30
RUSSIAN TWIST	0:30
SIDE BEND (LEFT)	0:30

MIND THE GAP

LEVEL 1 OR LEVEL 2

SET 1 (3 ROUNDS)	WORK
SPRINT	0:30
CROSS JACK	0:30
SEAL JACK	0:30
MOUNTAIN CLIMBER	0:30

SET 2 (3 ROUNDS)	WORK
SQUAT	0:30
REVERSE LUNGE	0:30
SQUAT HOLD	0:30
LATERAL LUNGE	0:30

SET 3 (3 ROUNDS)	WORK
PLANK	0:30
T-STAND (LEFT)	0:30
T-STAND (RIGHT)	0:30
THE MUMMY	0:30

SET 4 (3 ROUNDS)	WORK
HIGH KNEES	0:30
PUSH-UP	0:30
PIKE	0:30
BICYCLE CRUNCH	0:30

FLIRTY THIRTIES

TOTAL TIME: 30:00

Perform each set three times before moving to the next. Rest for 30 seconds between sets.

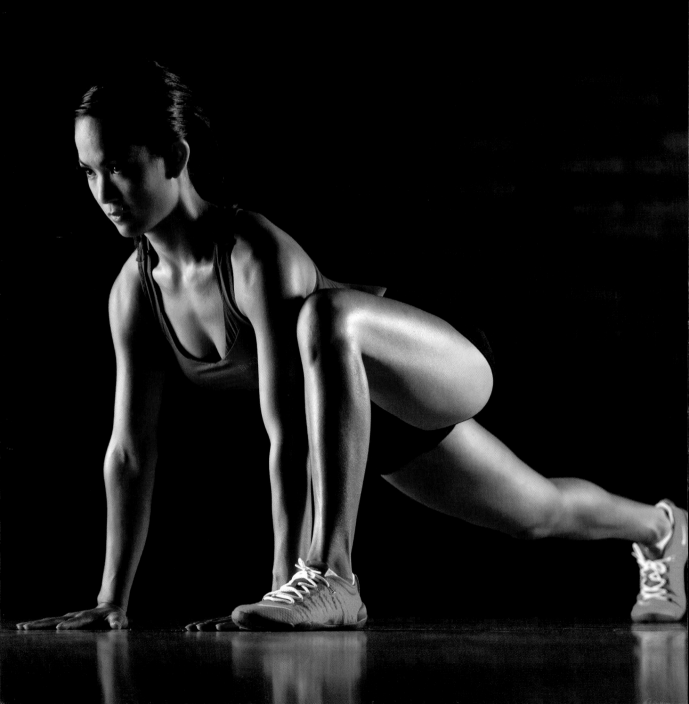

WHEN IN DOUBT WORKOUT

LEVEL 2 OR LEVEL 3

SET 1 (3 ROUNDS)	WORK
SPRINT	0:30
X-JACK	0:30
SEAL JACK	0:30
MOUNTAIN CLIMBER	0:30

SET 2 (3 ROUNDS)	WORK
SQUAT	0:30
REVERSE LUNGE	0:30
SQUAT JUMP	0:30
JUMP LUNGE	0:30

SET 3 (3 ROUNDS)	WORK
PLANK PUNCH	0:30
SPEED SKATER	0:30
MOGUL JUMP	0:30
STAR	0:30

SET 4 (3 ROUNDS)	WORK
HIGH KNEES	0:30
1-2 PUSH	0:30
PIKE	0:30
DOUBLE CROSS	0:30

FIT FRENZY

LEVEL 3

SET 1 (3 ROUNDS)	WORK
HIGH KNEES	0:30
GRASSHOPPER	0:30
BURPEE	0:30
SPIDERMAN	0:30

SET 2 (3 ROUNDS)	WORK
STAR	0:30
BALL PRESS	0:30
JUMP LUNGE	0:30
REACH	0:30

SET 3 (3 ROUNDS)	WORK
SIDE SUICIDES	0:30
SQUAT PEDAL	0:30
SKI JUMP	0:30
SPHINX	0:30

SET 4 (3 ROUNDS)	WORK
POWER KNEE (RIGHT)	0:30
SQUAT JUMP	0:30
POWER KNEE (LEFT)	0:30
1-2 PUSH	0:30

POWER HOUR 1

LEVEL 2 OR LEVEL 3

The appeal of most HIIT routines is that they're over quickly, but they don't have to be. If you're ready to take on a full hour of HIIT, this is for you. Do 10 minutes of dynamic stretching before beginning the cardio warm up.

WARM UP

Before you give it all you've got for the main workout, get your heart pumping with a quick cardio warm up. Start off nice and easy; you don't need to push to the max yet.

	WORK
SPRINT	0:30
JUMPING JACK	0:30
CROSS JACK	0:30
HIGH KNEES	0:30
SQUAT	0:30

REPEAT TWO TIMES.
TOTAL TIME: 5:00

WORKOUT

This is the main event. Push yourself as hard as possible for 45 minutes of fat burning, strength building, muscle toning work.

DO EACH SET THREE TIMES. REST FOR 30 SECONDS AFTER EACH SET.
TOTAL TIME: 45:00

SET 1	WORK	REST
SPRINT	0:30	0:00
SEAL JACK	0:30	0:00
MOUNTAIN CLIMBER	0:30	0:00
SKATER JUMP	0:30	0:00

SET 2	WORK	REST
CROSS-COUNTRY SEAL	0:30	0:00
BURPEE	0:30	0:00
SKI JUMP	0:30	0:00
STAR	0:30	0:00

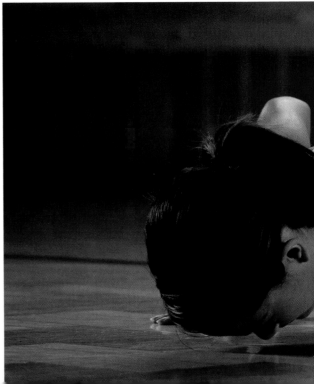

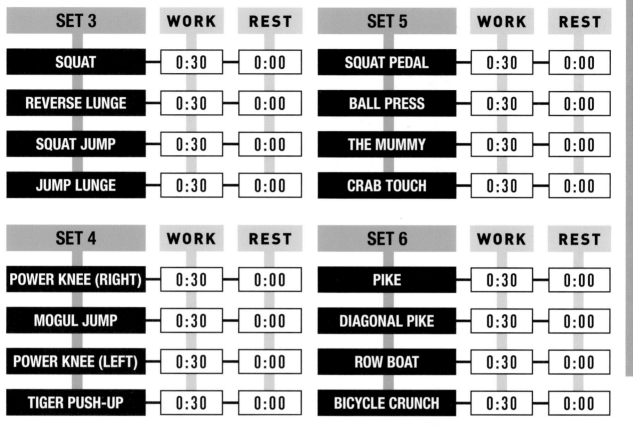

SET 3	WORK	REST
SQUAT	0:30	0:00
REVERSE LUNGE	0:30	0:00
SQUAT JUMP	0:30	0:00
JUMP LUNGE	0:30	0:00

SET 5	WORK	REST
SQUAT PEDAL	0:30	0:00
BALL PRESS	0:30	0:00
THE MUMMY	0:30	0:00
CRAB TOUCH	0:30	0:00

SET 4	WORK	REST
POWER KNEE (RIGHT)	0:30	0:00
MOGUL JUMP	0:30	0:00
POWER KNEE (LEFT)	0:30	0:00
TIGER PUSH-UP	0:30	0:00

SET 6	WORK	REST
PIKE	0:30	0:00
DIAGONAL PIKE	0:30	0:00
ROW BOAT	0:30	0:00
BICYCLE CRUNCH	0:30	0:00

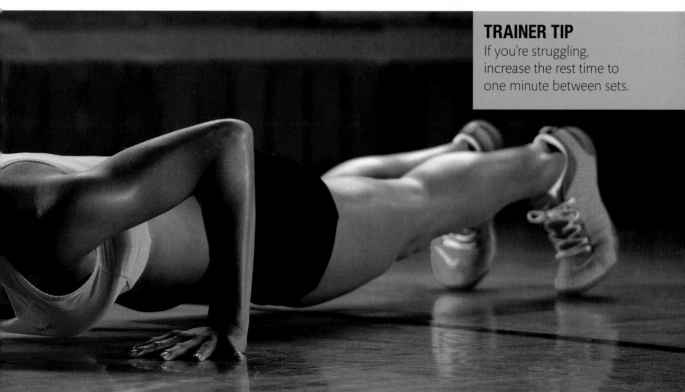

TRAINER TIP
If you're struggling, increase the rest time to one minute between sets.

POWER HOUR 2

LEVEL 2 OR LEVEL 3

Who said you need to keep it short and sweet? Prepare to burn over 800 calories with this grueling, hour-long workout. Be sure to do 10 minutes of dynamic stretching before beginning the cardio warm up.

WARM UP

Start things off with a quick cardio warm up. Don't push yourself yet; you should be working at 50 to 75 percent of your power.

	WORK
SPRINT	0:30
JUMPING JACK	0:30
HIGH KNEES	0:30
THE MUMMY	0:30
SQUAT	0:30

REPEAT TWO TIMES.
TOTAL TIME: 5:00

WORKOUT

Now it's time to kick it into high gear. Dig deep and keep your goals in mind.

DO EACH SET THREE TIMES. REST FOR 30 SECONDS AFTER EACH SET.
TOTAL TIME: 45:00

SET 1	WORK	REST
HIGH KNEES	0:30	0:00
1-2 PUSH	0:30	0:00
POWER KNEE (RIGHT)	0:30	0:00
POWER KNEE (LEFT)	0:30	0:00

SET 2	WORK	REST
SKI SQUAT	0:30	0:00
ALTERNATING LEG LIFT BURPEE	0:30	0:00
SKI JUMP	0:30	0:00
STAR	0:30	0:00

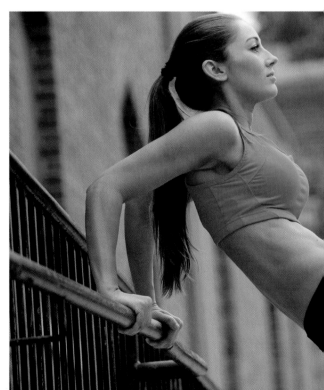

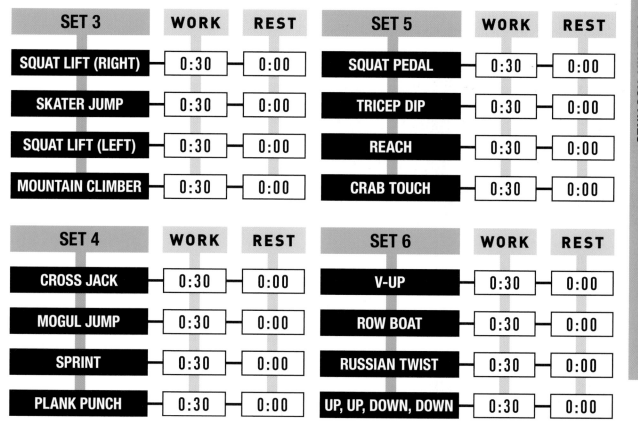

SET 3	WORK	REST
SQUAT LIFT (RIGHT)	0:30	0:00
SKATER JUMP	0:30	0:00
SQUAT LIFT (LEFT)	0:30	0:00
MOUNTAIN CLIMBER	0:30	0:00

SET 5	WORK	REST
SQUAT PEDAL	0:30	0:00
TRICEP DIP	0:30	0:00
REACH	0:30	0:00
CRAB TOUCH	0:30	0:00

SET 4	WORK	REST
CROSS JACK	0:30	0:00
MOGUL JUMP	0:30	0:00
SPRINT	0:30	0:00
PLANK PUNCH	0:30	0:00

SET 6	WORK	REST
V-UP	0:30	0:00
ROW BOAT	0:30	0:00
RUSSIAN TWIST	0:30	0:00
UP, UP, DOWN, DOWN	0:30	0:00

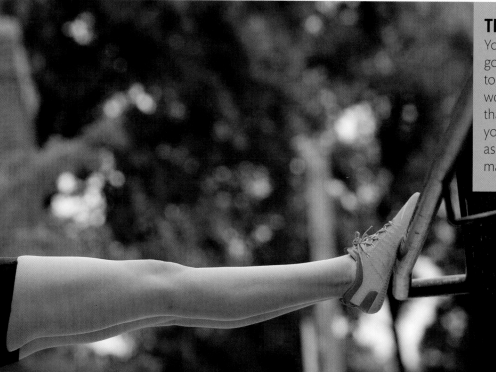

TRAINER TIP

Your mind and body are going to scream at you to stop during this workout. Remember that you get out what you put in. Push as hard as possible to get maximum results.

POWER HOUR 3

LEVEL 2 OR LEVEL 3

How long can you keep up the intensity? This hour-long workout will challenge your strength and endurance. To keep your muscles loose and limber, do 10 minutes of dynamic stretching before beginning the cardio warm up.

WARM UP

A five-minute cardio warm up will get your heart rate up before you take on the main workout. Take it easy on these exercises. You don't need to give it all you've got yet.

	WORK
SPRINT	0:30
CROSS JACK	0:30
HIGH KNEES	0:30
THE MUMMY	0:30
SQUAT	0:30

REPEAT TWO TIMES.
TOTAL TIME: 5:00

WORKOUT

Your warm up is over; now is the time to push yourself to the limit. Focus on form and don't let yourself slack. Do each exercise with purpose and intention.

DO EACH SET THREE TIMES. REST FOR 30 SECONDS AFTER EACH SET.
TOTAL TIME: 45:00

SET 1	WORK	REST
JUMPING JACK	0:30	0:00
ALTERNATING LEG LIFT BURPEE	0:30	0:00
SPRINT	0:30	0:00
1-2 PUSH	0:30	0:00

SET 2	WORK	REST
X-JACK	0:30	0:00
GRASSHOPPER	0:30	0:00
STAR	0:30	0:00
IN-AND-OUT ABS	0:30	0:00

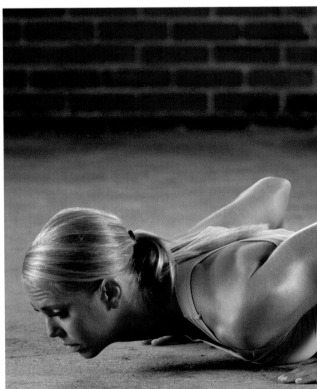

SET 3	WORK	REST
MOUNTAIN CLIMBER	0:30	0:00
TIGER PUSH-UP	0:30	0:00
JUMP LUNGE	0:30	0:00
MOGUL JUMP	0:30	0:00

SET 5	WORK	REST
4 CALF RAISES + 4 TAPS	0:30	0:00
CRAB TOUCH	0:30	0:00
THE MUMMY	0:30	0:00
CROSS PUSH	0:30	0:00

SET 4	WORK	REST
SKI SQUAT	0:30	0:00
LATERAL LUNGE	0:30	0:00
SHOULDER PRESS JACK	0:30	0:00
SQUAT PEDAL	0:30	0:00

SET 6	WORK	REST
POWER KNEE (RIGHT)	0:30	0:00
PLANK PUNCH	0:30	0:00
POWER KNEE (LEFT)	0:30	0:00
PLANK ROTATION	0:30	0:00

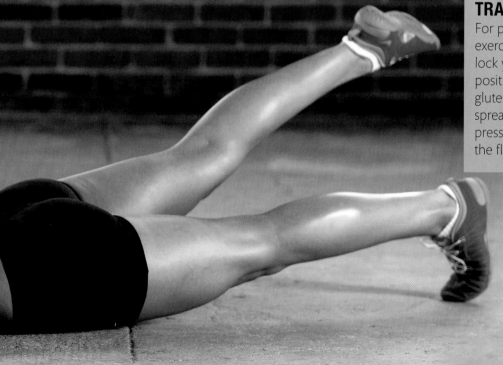

TRAINER TIP

For plank-based exercises, be sure to lock your body in position. Squeeze your glutes and quads, spread your fingers, and press your palms into the floor.

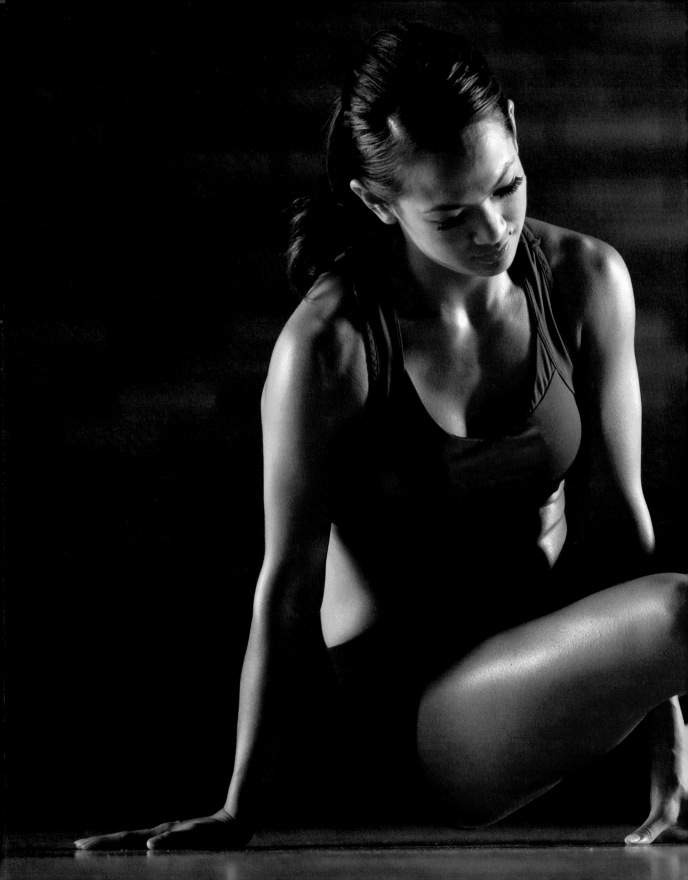

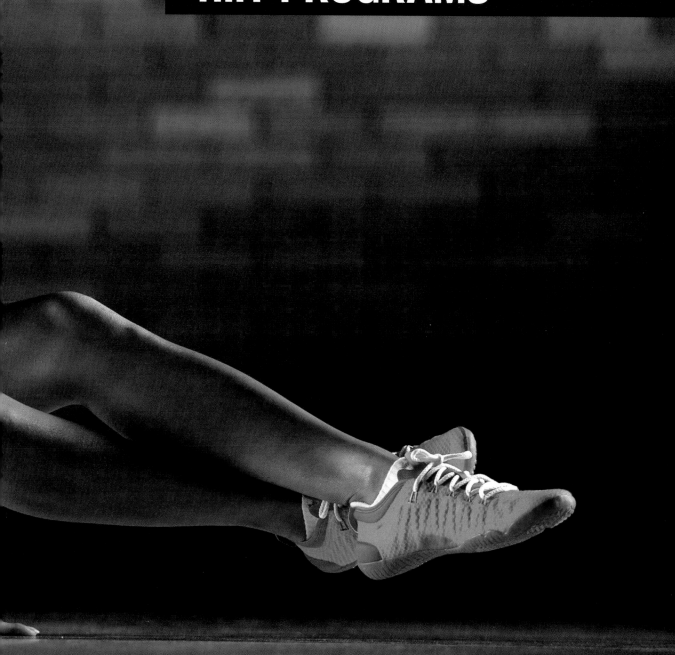

05

HIIT PROGRAMS

HIIT PROGRAMS

If you need more guidance in your HIIT journey, commit to taking a HIIT challenge. Whether you want to get started with a workout schedule, need a plan for which routines to follow, or are ready to take on 28 days of HIIT, there's a program for you.

3-Day Challenge
7-Day Challenge
14-Day Challenge
28-Day Challenge

Each program gives you a structured series of HIIT routines specifically chosen to maximize results. Choose a program that fits with your schedule, and challenge yourself to commit to HIIT for the duration.

THE 3-DAY CHALLENGE

This short but seductive introduction to HIIT is designed to leave you wanting more. If you do HIIT for just three days, you'll find it's much easier to make it part of your regular lifestyle. Each head-to-toe workout combines high-output cardio and compound strength exercises to give you a firm foundation for HIIT.

LEVEL 1

If you are having trouble getting started with HIIT, challenge yourself to three days of workouts that include some popular HIIT basics.

LEVELS 2 AND 3

If you are already at a high level of fitness and want to shake up your normal routine, this is a fun, energetic way to infuse some intensity into your workouts.

| DAY 1 | **JUST DO HIIT** | Start off with a routine centered on three of HIIT's bodyweight basics. This whole-body workout is a great way to formally introduce you to HIIT. |

| DAY 2 | **HEAD TO TONE** | Build on what you accomplished on Day 1. This routine introduces plyometrics and alternates between high-energy cardio and explosive strength-building exercises. |

| DAY 3 | **METABOLIC MAYHEM** | Day 3 brings your biggest challenge yet. HIIT is all about burning calories and pushing as hard as you can to maximize the post HIIT calorie after burn. Train insane or remain the same! |

TIPS

To decrease the risk of injury and prepare yourself to perform at 100 percent, remember to warm up each day before beginning your HIIT routine.

Focus on form before speed. Make sure you know how to do each exercise properly before beginning your routine.

Stay hydrated and don't let your diet undo all your hard work! To get the results you want, you'll need to work hard and eat right.

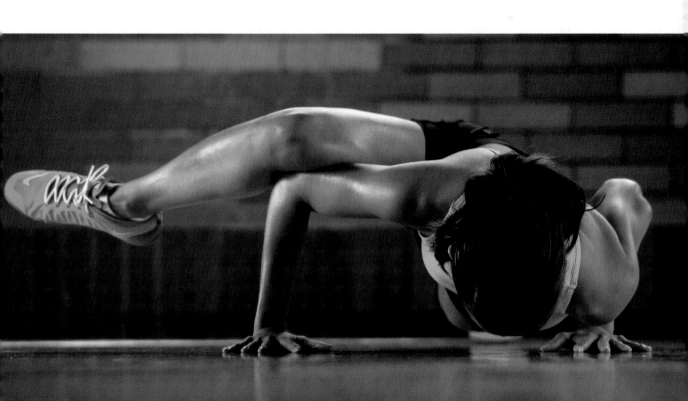

THE 7-DAY CHALLENGE

Looking to drop up to five pounds in seven days? Need to inject a little fire into your regular workout regime? The 7-Day Challenge introduces some new HIIT routine formats and features exercises designed to burn fat, lose weight, increase strength, and improve athletic performance.

LEVEL 1

Build a strong foundation from the ground up. The 7-Day Challenge includes plyometrics and strength-building exercises, as well as routines that focus on the legs and core.

LEVELS 2 AND 3

Routines featuring a blend of short and long sets, plyometrics, compound strength exercises, and core-building exercises will kick your workouts into high gear. Give it all you've got, and you'll be amazed at the results you can achieve in just seven days.

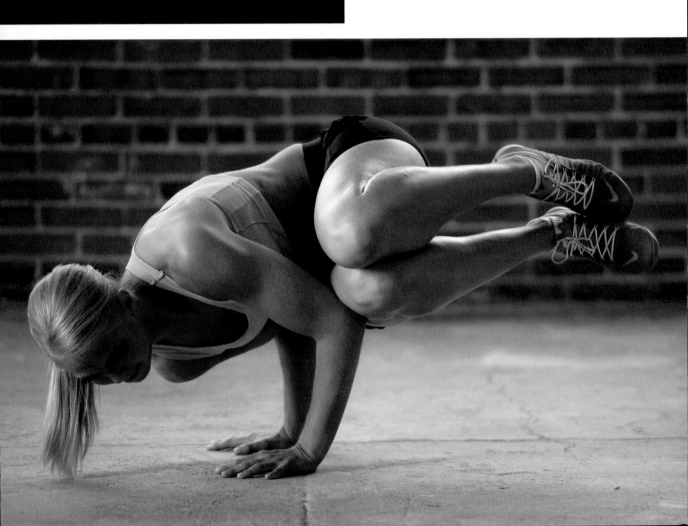

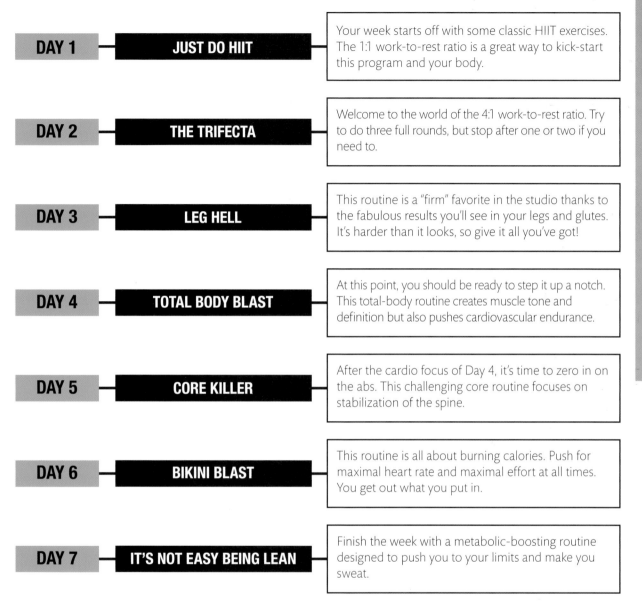

DAY 1	JUST DO HIIT	Your week starts off with some classic HIIT exercises. The 1:1 work-to-rest ratio is a great way to kick-start this program and your body.
DAY 2	THE TRIFECTA	Welcome to the world of the 4:1 work-to-rest ratio. Try to do three full rounds, but stop after one or two if you need to.
DAY 3	LEG HELL	This routine is a "firm" favorite in the studio thanks to the fabulous results you'll see in your legs and glutes. It's harder than it looks, so give it all you've got!
DAY 4	TOTAL BODY BLAST	At this point, you should be ready to step it up a notch. This total-body routine creates muscle tone and definition but also pushes cardiovascular endurance.
DAY 5	CORE KILLER	After the cardio focus of Day 4, it's time to zero in on the abs. This challenging core routine focuses on stabilization of the spine.
DAY 6	BIKINI BLAST	This routine is all about burning calories. Push for maximal heart rate and maximal effort at all times. You get out what you put in.
DAY 7	IT'S NOT EASY BEING LEAN	Finish the week with a metabolic-boosting routine designed to push you to your limits and make you sweat.

TIPS

To perform your best and prevent injury, begin each routine with a three- to five-minute warm up.

The 7-Day Challenge introduces more athletic exercises, so form is more important than ever. Be sure you know how to do each exercise correctly before beginning your routine.

Expect to be sore. If your workouts are as intense as they should be, you will be sore the next day. Remember that sore muscles are not the same as pain due to injury.

This program was designed to be undertaken on back-to-back days, but if necessary, you can take a rest day between workouts. Listen to your body and allow the appropriate recovery time.

THE 14-DAY CHALLENGE

If you're willing to commit to two weeks of HIIT, you'll be able to see a change in your body. The routines in this program will help you lose weight, build strength, and improve cardiovascular endurance with a combination of body weight and plyometric exercises. The 14-Day Challenge incorporates focused routines for the core and lower body to break up the high-impact routines and ensure you can give 100 percent each and every day.

LEVEL 1

As you progress from Day 1 to Day 14, the routines will become more difficult, challenging you even as your strength and fitness increase. Pay attention to form and push yourself to work harder each day.

LEVELS 2 AND 3

The challenge is even greater at Levels 2 and 3. This program includes three hour-long routines, which require you to put forth your greatest effort for an extended period of time.

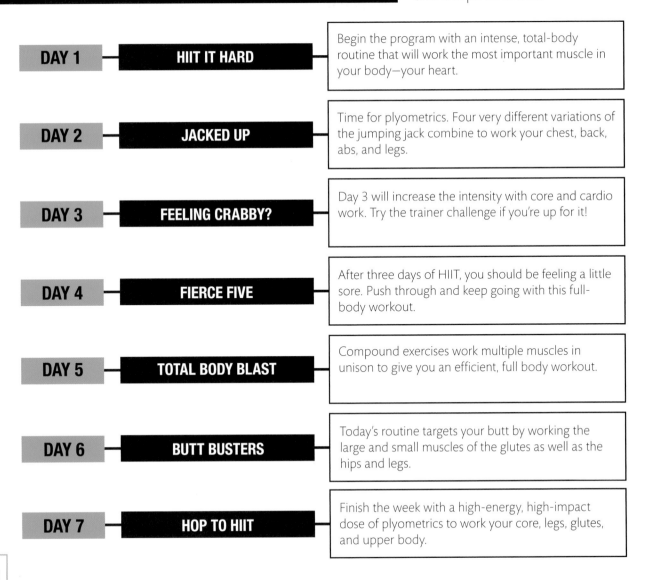

DAY 1 — HIIT IT HARD
Begin the program with an intense, total-body routine that will work the most important muscle in your body—your heart.

DAY 2 — JACKED UP
Time for plyometrics. Four very different variations of the jumping jack combine to work your chest, back, abs, and legs.

DAY 3 — FEELING CRABBY?
Day 3 will increase the intensity with core and cardio work. Try the trainer challenge if you're up for it!

DAY 4 — FIERCE FIVE
After three days of HIIT, you should be feeling a little sore. Push through and keep going with this full-body workout.

DAY 5 — TOTAL BODY BLAST
Compound exercises work multiple muscles in unison to give you an efficient, full body workout.

DAY 6 — BUTT BUSTERS
Today's routine targets your butt by working the large and small muscles of the glutes as well as the hips and legs.

DAY 7 — HOP TO HIIT
Finish the week with a high-energy, high-impact dose of plyometrics to work your core, legs, glutes, and upper body.

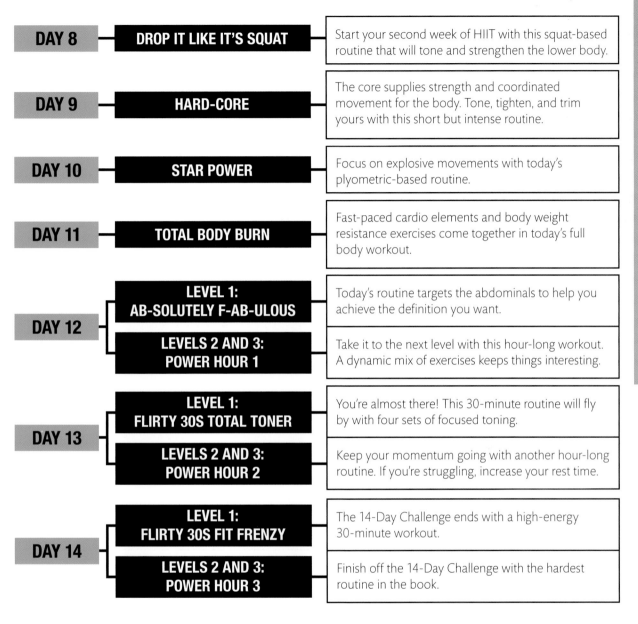

DAY 8	**DROP IT LIKE IT'S SQUAT**	Start your second week of HIIT with this squat-based routine that will tone and strengthen the lower body.
DAY 9	**HARD-CORE**	The core supplies strength and coordinated movement for the body. Tone, tighten, and trim yours with this short but intense routine.
DAY 10	**STAR POWER**	Focus on explosive movements with today's plyometric-based routine.
DAY 11	**TOTAL BODY BURN**	Fast-paced cardio elements and body weight resistance exercises come together in today's full body workout.
DAY 12	**LEVEL 1:** **AB-SOLUTELY F-AB-ULOUS**	Today's routine targets the abdominals to help you achieve the definition you want.
	LEVELS 2 AND 3: **POWER HOUR 1**	Take it to the next level with this hour-long workout. A dynamic mix of exercises keeps things interesting.
DAY 13	**LEVEL 1:** **FLIRTY 30S TOTAL TONER**	You're almost there! This 30-minute routine will fly by with four sets of focused toning.
	LEVELS 2 AND 3: **POWER HOUR 2**	Keep your momentum going with another hour-long routine. If you're struggling, increase your rest time.
DAY 14	**LEVEL 1:** **FLIRTY 30S FIT FRENZY**	The 14-Day Challenge ends with a high-energy 30-minute workout.
	LEVELS 2 AND 3: **POWER HOUR 3**	Finish off the 14-Day Challenge with the hardest routine in the book.

TIPS

Remember that quality is more important than quantity. The 14-Day Challenge introduces more athletic exercises, which means attention to form is critical.

Stay mentally strong and focus on your goals. Two weeks takes dedication. It's easy for "just one day off" to turn into two and then three. Stick with it.

Be aware of what you eat. You'll see greater changes if you are disciplined in your eating as well as your exercise.

A number of the routines in this program include a "Trainer Challenge." If you're up for it, tackle these instead of the traditional routines.

Assess your fitness at the start of the two-week program and at the end. By Day 14, you should see results!

THE 28-DAY CHALLENGE

When the Indianapolis Colts Cheerleaders need to prepare for a swimsuit calendar shoot, this is the program they use. It will help you burn fat, lose weight, and tone your body while making you stronger and more athletic. As the weeks progress, the routines become more challenging, adapting to your increasing strength and fitness. The variety of routine styles and formats will keep your body on its toes and give you the results you want.

LEVEL 1

The goal of the 28-Day Challenge is to get you strong and confident enough during the first 14 days to transition to Level 2 for the last two weeks. Stick to the workout plan, assess your fitness, and take it to the next level.

LEVELS 2 AND 3

This four-week program is designed to take you to your peak level of fitness. Don't slack off; keep pushing yourself to do more during each "work" interval. The more you put in, the more you'll get out.

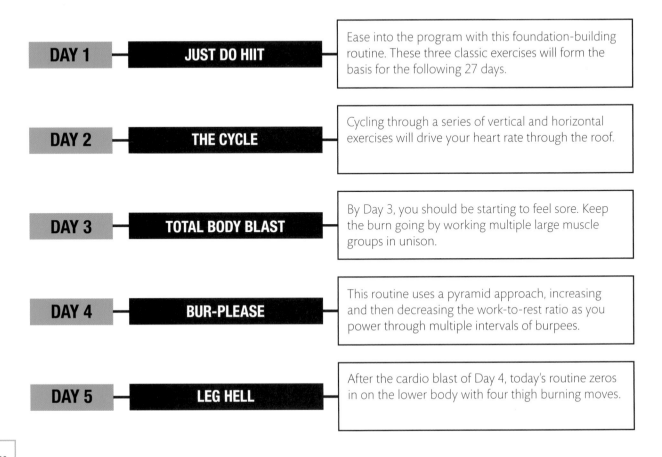

DAY 1 — **JUST DO HIIT**

Ease into the program with this foundation-building routine. These three classic exercises will form the basis for the following 27 days.

DAY 2 — **THE CYCLE**

Cycling through a series of vertical and horizontal exercises will drive your heart rate through the roof.

DAY 3 — **TOTAL BODY BLAST**

By Day 3, you should be starting to feel sore. Keep the burn going by working multiple large muscle groups in unison.

DAY 4 — **BUR-PLEASE**

This routine uses a pyramid approach, increasing and then decreasing the work-to-rest ratio as you power through multiple intervals of burpees.

DAY 5 — **LEG HELL**

After the cardio blast of Day 4, today's routine zeros in on the lower body with four thigh burning moves.

DAY 6 — **THE TRIFECTA**

A 4:1 work-to-rest ratio means intense fat burning. Get ready to sweat with a workout that will challenge every facet of your fitness.

DAY 7 — **FLIRTY 30S MIND THE GAP**

Finish the week with a 30-minute, total-body challenge. Dig deep, push hard, and give it all you can.

DAY 8 — **TOTAL BODY BURN**

This routine gets your second week off to an explosive start with a combination of cardio and compound exercises to make it burn!

DAY 9 — **"T" IT UP**

Day 9 brings the intensity down a notch to allow for unilateral training, improving balance, coordination, and mobility.

DAY 10 — **ROW NO YOU DON'T**

The three core exercises in this routine activate the upper and lower body simultaneously.

DAY 11 — **HEAD TO TONE**

Push your cardiovascular endurance with a longer routine alternating between high-energy cardio and athletic exercises.

DAY 12 — **BUTT BUSTERS**

Slow the pace today to focus on the hips, glutes, and legs. The slower pace doesn't mean it's easy; your butt will feel the burn.

DAY 13 — **BIKINI BLAST**

Today's fast-paced workout focuses on cardio and core work to burn fat and tone your abs.

DAY 14 — **FLIRTY 30S FIT FRENZY**

Halfway there! After two weeks of HIIT, you should be feeling stronger and leaner. Keep it going with this fast-paced, 30-minute workout.

THE 28-DAY CHALLENGE

DAY 15 — **FIERCE FIVE**

Your third week begins with a routine designed to push your heart rate through the roof. Don't forget to reassess your fitness!

DAY 16 — **FEELING CRABBY?**

You may be feeling crabby and ready for a break, but stick to it! After this routine, you'll feel strong and energized.

DAY 17 — **FLIRTY 30S TOTAL TONER**

Kick up the intensity with this 30-minute, total-body workout.

DAY 18 — **STAR POWER**

Increase your speed and power with the plyometric exercises in this intense cardio workout.

DAY 19 — **IT'S NOT EASY BEING LEAN**

Boost your metabolism and your heart rate with three sets of total body exercises.

DAY 20 — **DROP IT LIKE IT'S SQUAT**

Today's routine will have your legs burning. Keep an eye on form, even when you get tired.

DAY 21 — **POWER HOUR 1**

Week three wraps up with an intense hour of HIIT. You can do this! Stay focused, determined, and committed.

DAY 22 — **FLIRTY 30S WHEN IN DOUBT, WORK OUT**

Get the last week of your 28-Day Challenge off to a strong start by pushing yourself to the limit during this 30-minute routine.

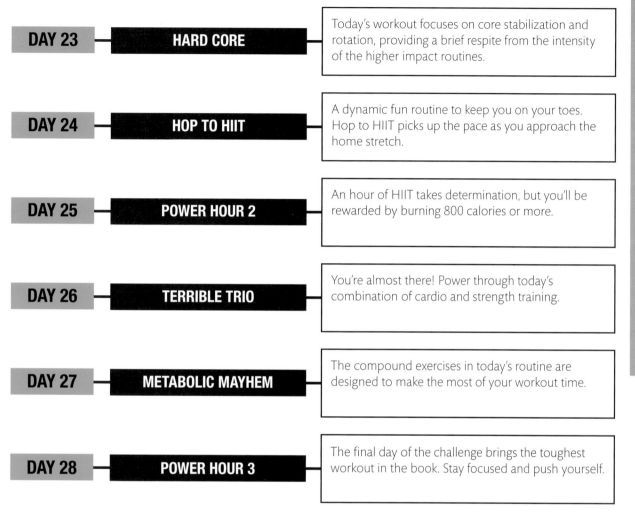

DAY 23 — **HARD CORE**

Today's workout focuses on core stabilization and rotation, providing a brief respite from the intensity of the higher impact routines.

DAY 24 — **HOP TO HIIT**

A dynamic fun routine to keep you on your toes. Hop to HIIT picks up the pace as you approach the home stretch.

DAY 25 — **POWER HOUR 2**

An hour of HIIT takes determination, but you'll be rewarded by burning 800 calories or more.

DAY 26 — **TERRIBLE TRIO**

You're almost there! Power through today's combination of cardio and strength training.

DAY 27 — **METABOLIC MAYHEM**

The compound exercises in today's routine are designed to make the most of your workout time.

DAY 28 — **POWER HOUR 3**

The final day of the challenge brings the toughest workout in the book. Stay focused and push yourself.

TIPS

Assess your fitness before beginning the 28-Day Challenge and again after Day 14. Adjust your workout level accordingly.

A number of the routines include an optional trainer challenge. Substitute these for the regular routine if you're looking for a tougher workout.

Setting aside a specific time for HIIT each day will make it easier to stay on track. Make a plan each week for your workouts and stick to it.

You will likely experience soreness if you haven't been working out regularly, especially during the first week. Take time to stretch and use a foam roller to aid in muscle recovery.

If you're making the commitment to do HIIT for 28 days, commit to monitoring your diet as well. Getting the results you want takes discipline.

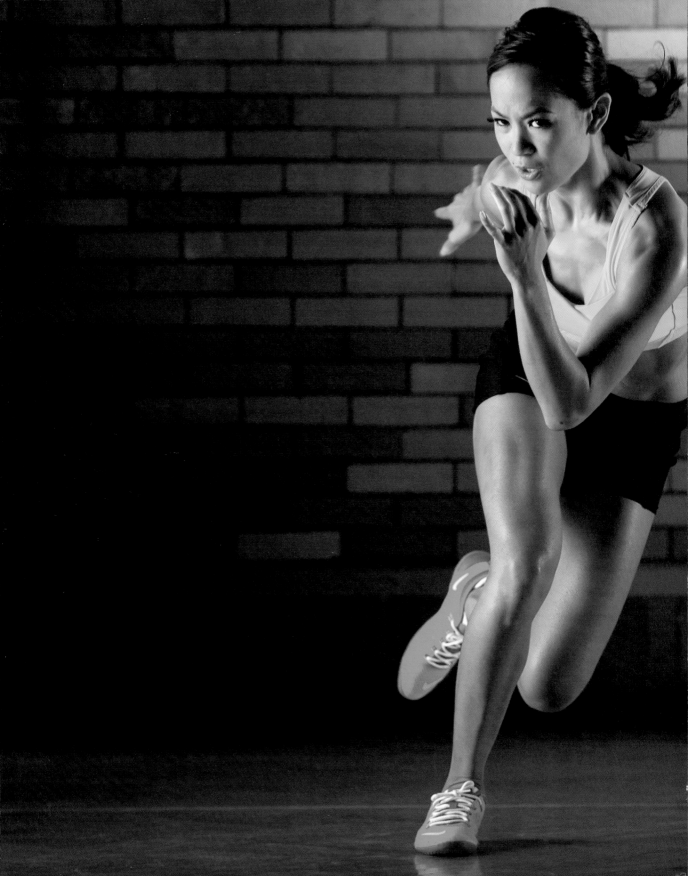

CARDIO EXERCISES

JUMPING JACK

There's a reason jumping jacks have long been a staple of high school gym class. This explosive move is a great way to improve cardiovascular endurance and also engage the core, shoulders, back, and calves.

TRAINER TIP
Try to remain in the "ready" position, on the balls of the feet with a soft bend in the knees.

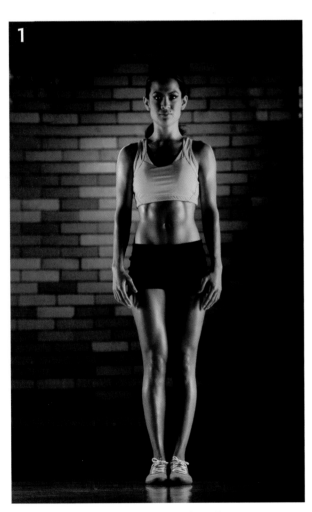

Stand with feet together and arms by sides. Engage the core and soften the knees.

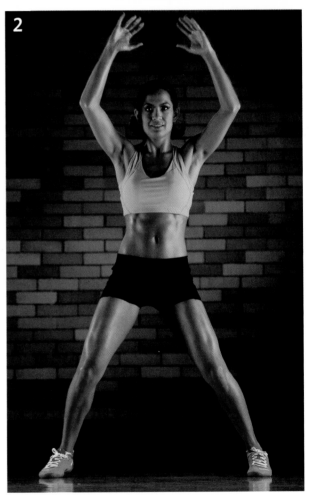

Jump up as you spread your feet wider than the shoulders and raise your arms overhead. Land with feet spread and arms up. Jump again, bringing your feet together and returning your arms to the sides. Repeat.

X-JACK

This innovative twist on the traditional jumping jack will boost your metabolism and tone your legs, core, shoulders, and back.

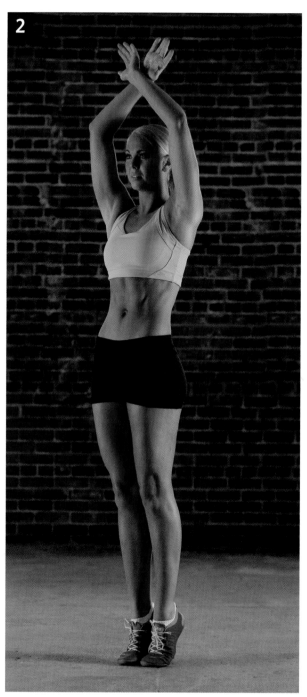

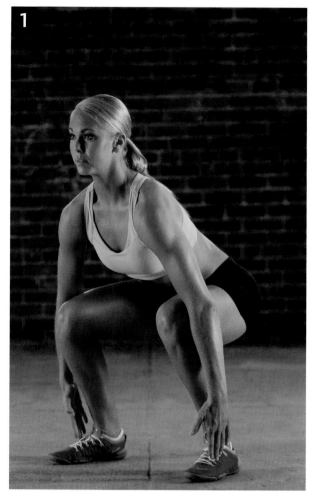

With feet shoulder-width apart, bend from your hips, knees, and ankles and drop into a squat position. If you can, touch your toes with your fingertips. Hold your chest up, look forward, and keep your weight in your heels.

Jump out of the squat position. As you jump, extend your legs and raise your arms overhead, crossing your wrists to make an X. Land with your feet together, weight on balls of feet. Keep a soft bend in your knees and engage the core.

BURPEE

The burpee is indisputably the ultimate total body exercise. Each one will work your chest, arms, shoulders, thighs, hamstrings, and core. Burpees can be intimidating, but the benefits are worth the challenge.

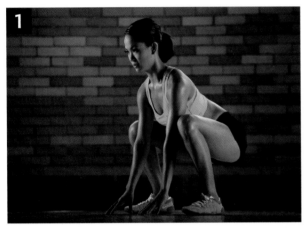

With your feet hip-width apart, bend your knees and bring hands to the floor just in front of your feet. Spread your fingers wide and grip the floor.

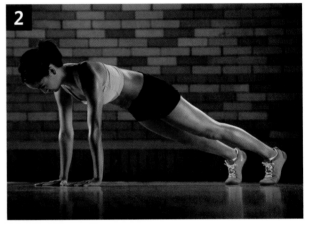

Hop your feet back into a plank position. Don't allow your lower back to collapse.

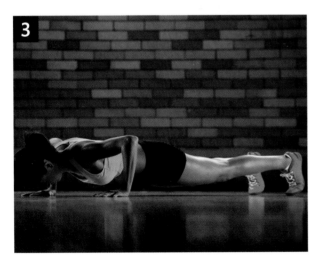

Perform one push-up with your core engaged.

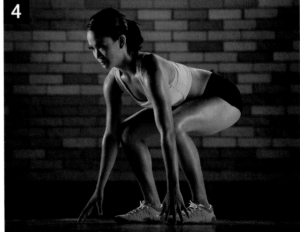

Jump your feet back to your hands, shifting your weight to the heels and lifting your chest.

CHALLENGE

For added challenge, substitute the regular push-up with a triceps push-up, keeping your elbows tight to your rib cage.

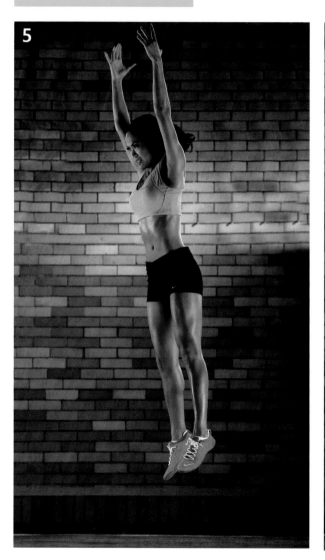

5

Jump up from the crouched position and reach overhead with your hands.

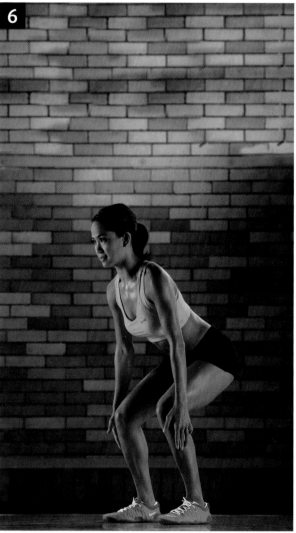

6

Land softly with a slight bend at your knees, hips, and ankles.

CROSS-COUNTRY SEAL

This exercise mimics the motion of cross-country skiing and improves cardiovascular endurance by working all the major muscle groups of the body. The cross-country seal opens the arms laterally, creating a multi-planar exercise that targets the shoulders, back, legs, and glutes.

TRAINER TIP
Try to always be in the "ready" position, on the balls of the feet with a soft bend in the knees.

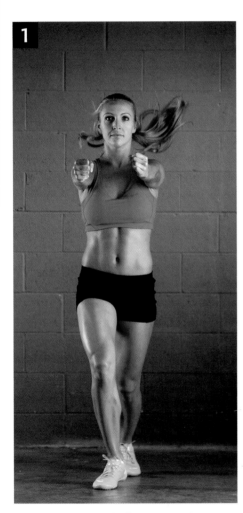

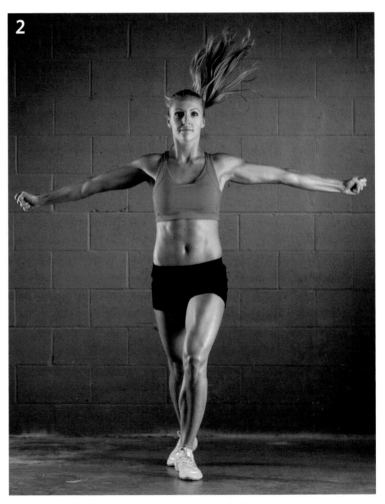

Stand with your right foot two to three feet in front of the left and extend your arms in front of the body. Keep a soft bend in your knees, engage your core, and lean forward slightly.

Jump and switch feet, opening your arms and squeezing your shoulder blades while in the air. Land softly, with your left foot in front of the right.

MOUNTAIN CLIMBER

The mountain climber challenges the stabilizing muscles of the core while kicking up your heart rate with rapid foot movement. Keep your feet moving quickly to maximize the burn.

CHALLENGE

Try elevating your hands on a small step, bench, or stability ball to increase the difficulty of this exercise.

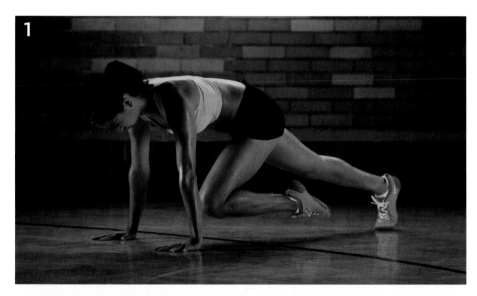

1

Position your hands on the floor slightly wider than shoulder-width apart. Rise up onto your toes and engage the core to form a straight line between your toes and head.

Bend your left leg and pull your knee in toward your chest, engaging your core.

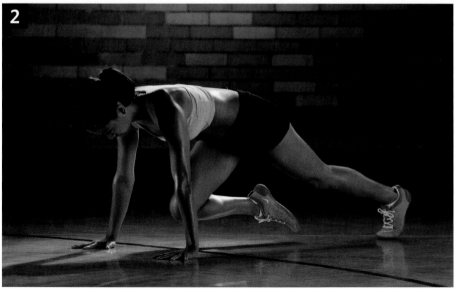

2

Extend the left leg and simultaneously pull the right knee toward the chest. Attempt to pull your knee all the way through your supporting arms to maximize the engagement of your core. Repeat with controlled speed.

ALTERNATING LEG LIFT BURPEE

The alternating leg lift burpee takes the traditional burpee and adds a leg lift for a challenging twist. Do this move as quickly as possible while maintaining proper form.

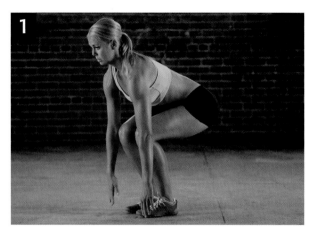

With your feet hip-distance apart, bend your knees and place your hands on the floor just in front of your feet.

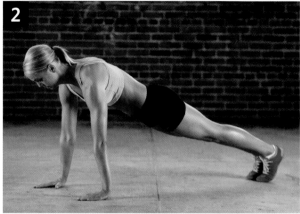

Hop back with both feet into a plank position.

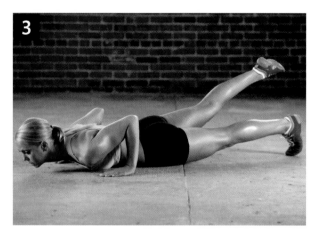

Perform a push-up. As you bend your arms, lift your right leg to hip height. Do not allow your back to arch when lifting your leg.

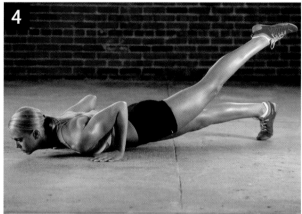

Return to the plank position and perform a second push-up. As you bend your arms, lift your left leg to hip height.

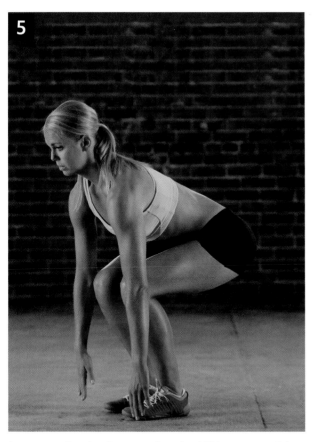

Jump your feet back to your hands, shifting your weight to your heels and lifting your chest.

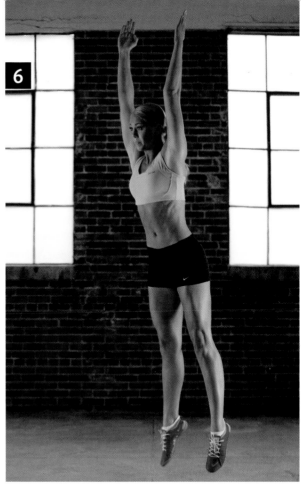

Jump from the crouched position, reaching overhead with your hands. Land softly with a slight bend in the knees, hips, and ankles.

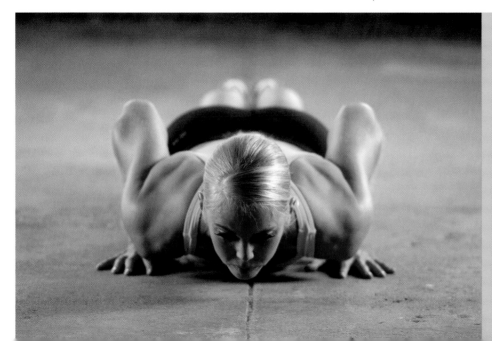

CHALLENGE

For added challenge, complete the movement in the triceps push-up position, with elbows tucked against rib cage.

GRASSHOPPER

The grasshopper's powerful legs are the inspiration for this exercise. This move will burn and firm the thighs, core, and shoulders while increasing athletic performance and hip mobility. Hop to it!

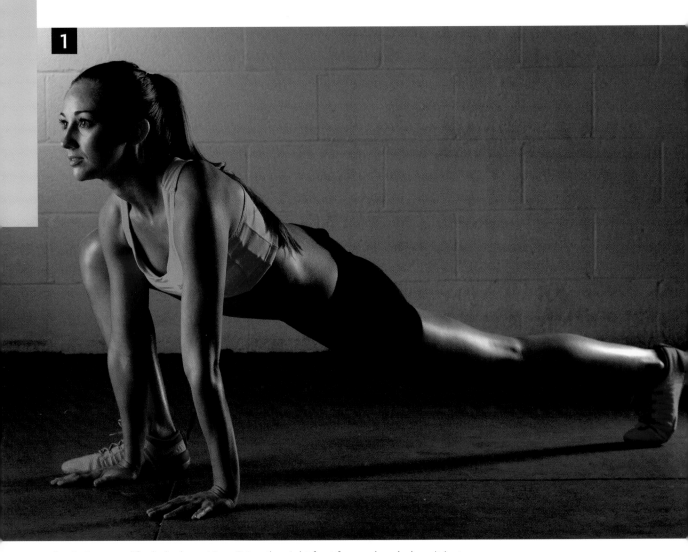

1

Begin in a modified plank position. Bring the right foot forward and place it just outside your right hand, bending the leg 90 degrees. Keep your body in a straight line from left foot to head.

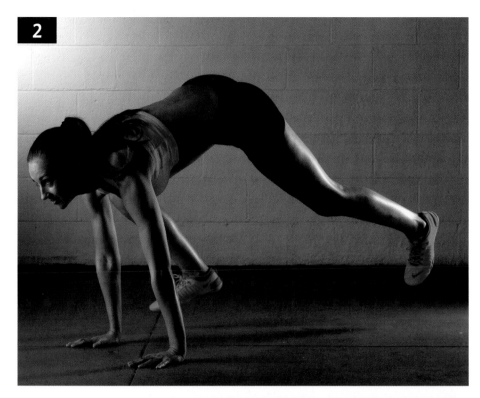

Jump and switch the feet.

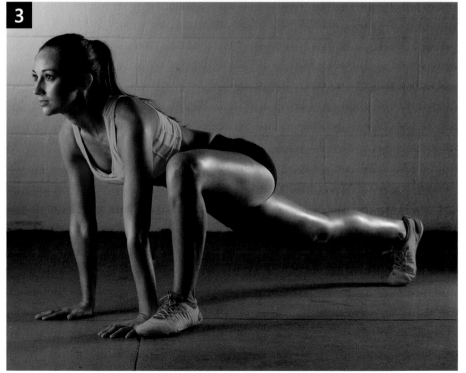

Land with the left foot on the floor on the outside of the left hand. Repeat, alternating legs with controlled speed.

SPRINT

Sprinting is a simple and effective means of elevating your heart rate and burning fat. This high-intensity exercise can be done in place or back and forth across an open space.

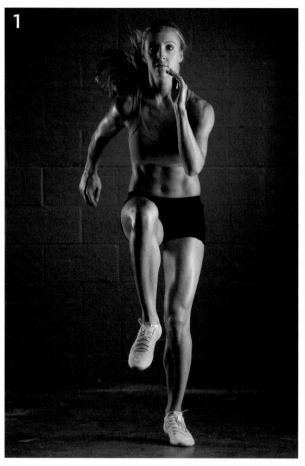

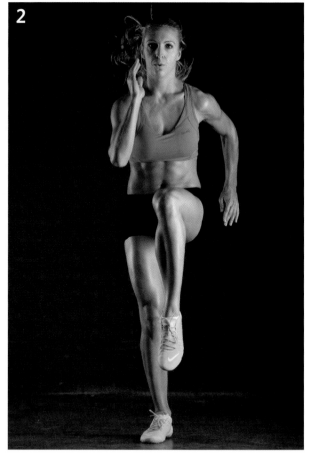

Stand tall, with feet shoulder-width apart and a slight lean to the body. Drive right knee to chest as left arm swings forward. Keep core engaged.

As your right leg lowers, drive forward with your left knee and right arm. Repeat with control, always moving opposite arms and legs.

CROSS JACK

This modified jumping jack requires coordination, balance, and stability. It will increase your heart rate, fire up your metabolism, and tone the shoulders, thighs, glutes, and hamstrings.

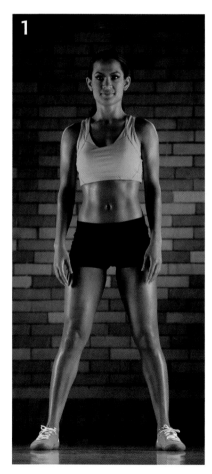

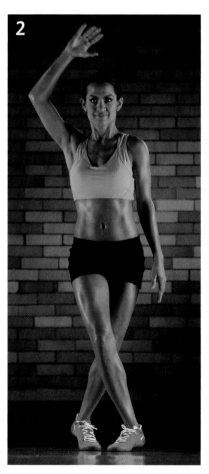

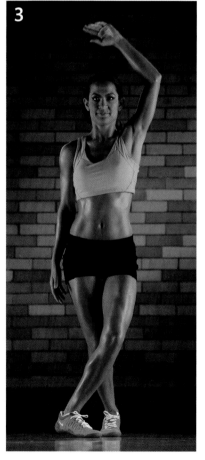

Stand with feet wider than your shoulders and arms at your sides. Softly bend the knees and engage the core.

Jump, landing with right foot crossed in front of left and right arm overhead.

Jump, this time landing with left foot crossed in front of right and left arm overhead.

HIGH KNEES

This is an excellent exercise for runners and athletes who want to improve running form and foot speed. The dynamic running motion will challenge your cardiovascular endurance and help to strengthen your hip flexors.

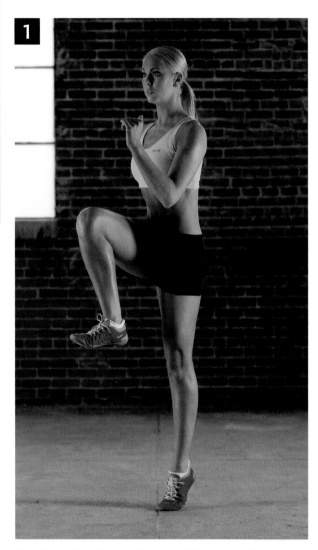

Stand with feet hip-width apart. Drive your right knee toward your chest and quickly place it back on the ground.

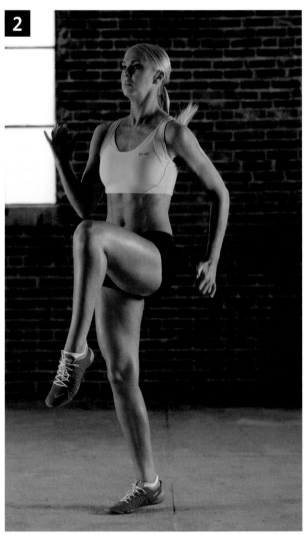

Immediately follow by driving the left knee to the chest. Alternate knees as quickly as you can. Bring your knees to your belly button or higher.

THE MUMMY

The mummy is a simple yet fun and highly effective way to charge your metabolism and tone your shoulders. Complete the move as quickly as possible for maximum benefit.

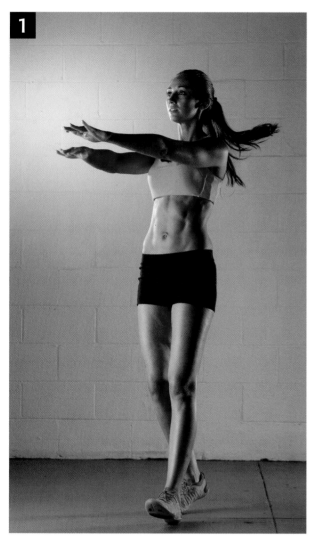

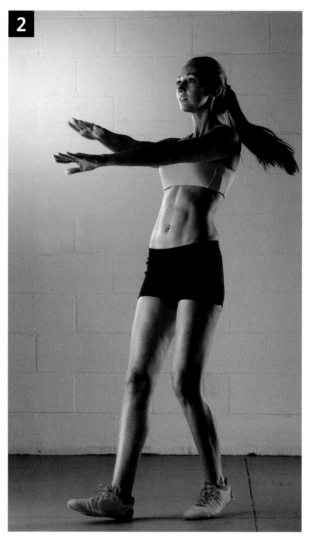

Stand with the heel of your left foot slightly in front of the right foot. Extend your arms in front of your chest and cross the left arm above the right. Keep your chin up and core engaged.

Jump, switching both feet and arms to land with the right heel in front of the left foot, right arm above left. Repeat at a fast but controlled pace.

SIDE SUICIDES

This whole-body exercise will not only amp up your heart rate, but will also improve your speed, coordination, and sports skills. The lateral shuffle works both the inner and outer thighs, and coordinated upper and lower body movements improve your athletic performance. Move as quickly as possible while maintaining proper form.

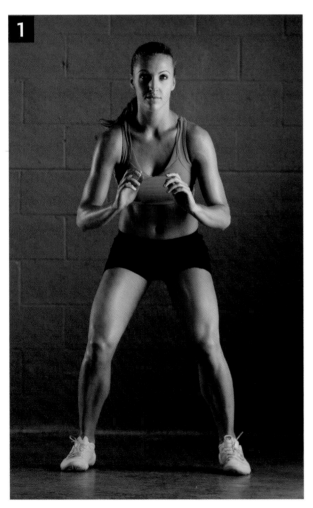

Bend hips and knees and sink into a mini-squat position. Lean forward slightly, but keep the back straight. This is the "ready" position.

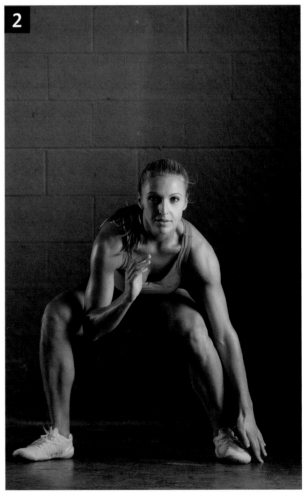

Shuffle two steps to the left. Sink deeper by bending at the hips, knees, and ankles. Reach down with the left hand to touch the floor.

CAUTION

Drop straight down to touch the floor. Don't lean out too far over one hip or reach beyond the outside of the foot. This could cause over pronation and lead to injury.

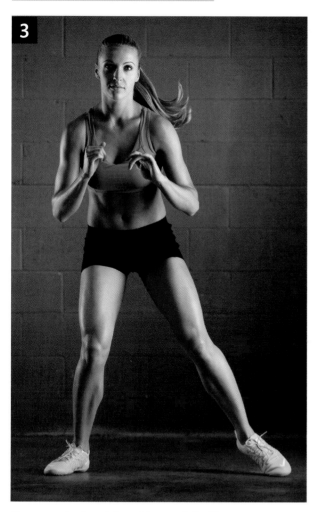

Return to the "ready" position and shuffle two steps to the right.

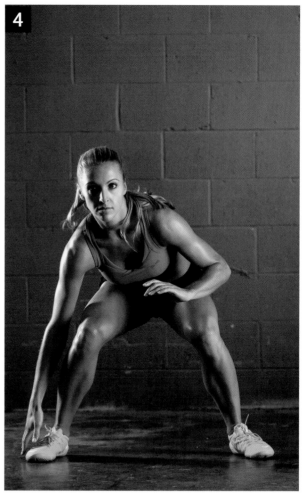

Sink into a deep squat and touch the floor with the right hand. Repeat, alternating sides.

SEAL JACK

This jumping jack variation involves opening and closing the arms for greater activation of the muscles in the back. Add seal jacks to your workout to get your back and shoulders toned.

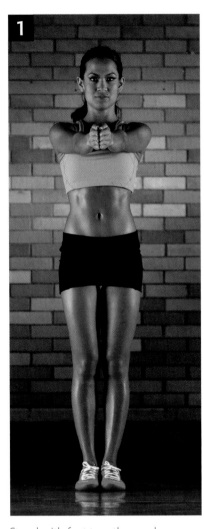

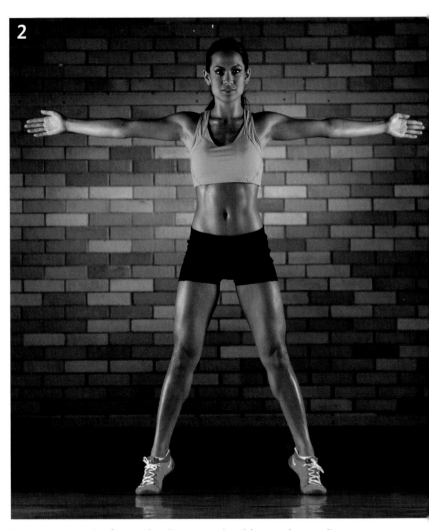

Stand with feet together and arms extended in front of your chest, palms together. Keep a soft bend at the knees and stay on the balls of your feet.

Jump, opening the feet wider than your shoulders and spreading your arms as wide as possible. Squeeze the muscles between the shoulder blades. Jump again, bringing the feet together as you clap your hands. Repeat.

MOGUL JUMP

The inspiration for this fat-blasting move comes from downhill skiing. Mogul jumps specifically target the lower abdominals and obliques, but also engage the shoulders, chest, hips, and thighs. Working all those muscles in unison makes your heart rate skyrocket and body fat percentage plummet.

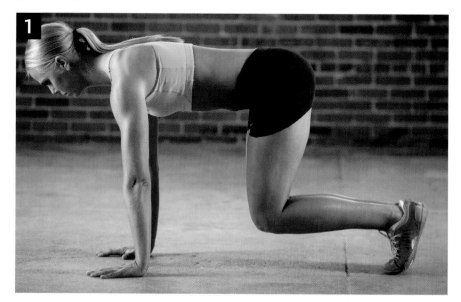

Begin on all fours with your arms straight and your legs together. Lift your knees off of the ground so that your legs are bent at a 90-degree angle and your weight is balanced between your hands and the balls of your feet. Your shins should be parallel to the floor.

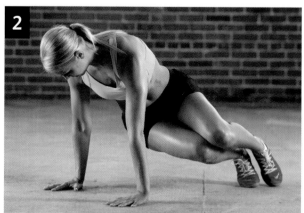

Keeping your arms straight and your knees together, hop and rotate your feet and knees to the left, rotating as much as possible. The knees should be perpendicular to the body and the hips in line with the shoulders.

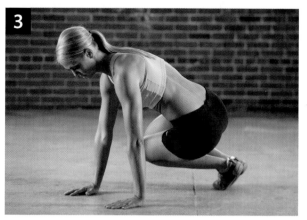

Jump and rotate feet and knees to the opposite side, keeping arms straight and knees together. Repeat, moving as quickly as possible while maintaining proper form.

POWER KNEE

This explosive movement is guaranteed to elevate your heart rate and make the abs, hip flexors, and thighs scream. Move as quickly as possible while maintaining proper form, and remember to do the same number of reps on each leg.

CAUTION
Keep your head up. You should be rotating your torso and bringing the knee across the body to the chest, not tucking the chin and rounding the spine.

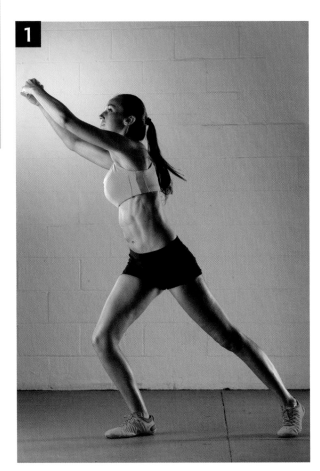

Stand tall with your feet slightly wider than your shoulders. Extend your arms straight overhead and interlace your fingers. Turn your body 45 degrees to the right, lifting the heel of your left foot.

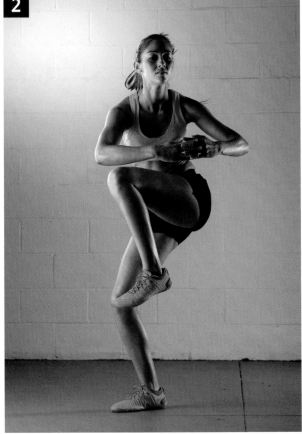

Bring the left knee up to the chest, driving it toward the right shoulder in an explosive motion, and simultaneously pull your arms down. Return to the starting position and repeat.

STAR

Who doesn't want to be a star? The squat jump meets the jumping jack in this plyometric powerhouse that will put you on the A-list.

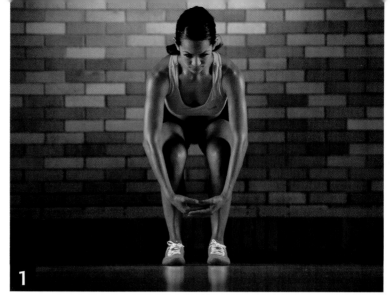

1

Stand tall, feet shoulder-width apart and toes pointing forward. With your body weight in your heels, inhale as you bend at the knee, lowering your body and wrapping your arms loosely around your shins.

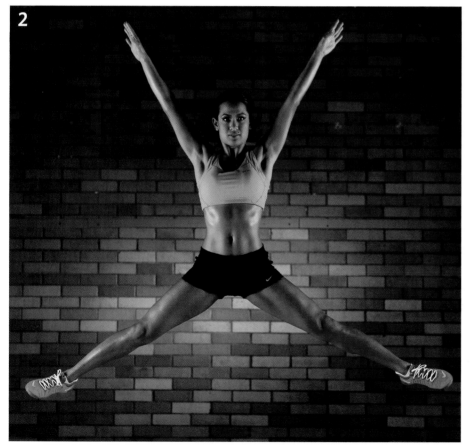

2

Engage your core and exhale as you jump and explode through your heels into the air. Open your arms and legs as wide as you can, making a "star" shape. Lengthen your entire body as you extend your arms and legs.

Land as softly and silently as possible, bending slightly at the hips, knees, and ankles to decelerate the body.

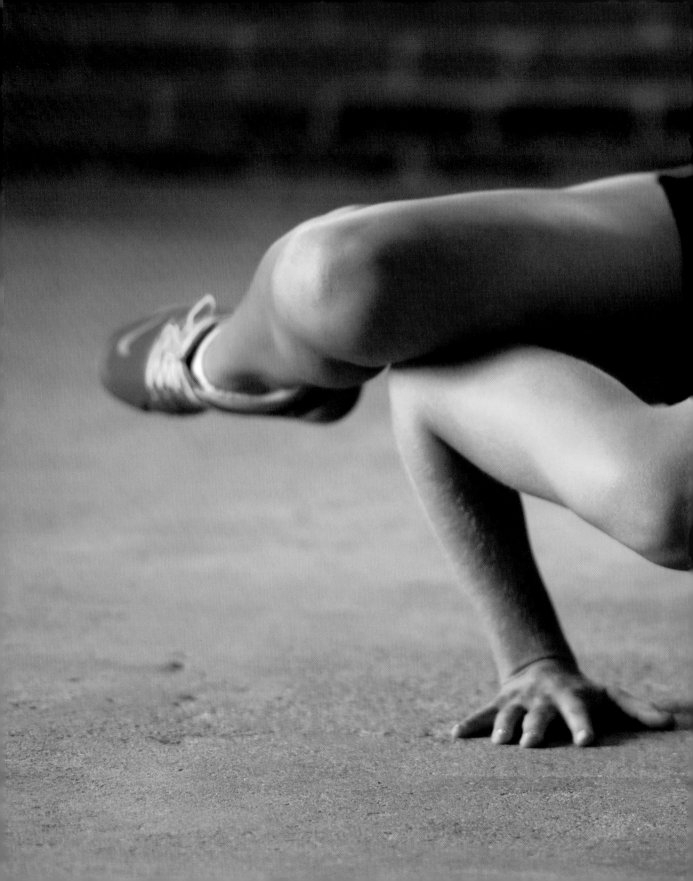

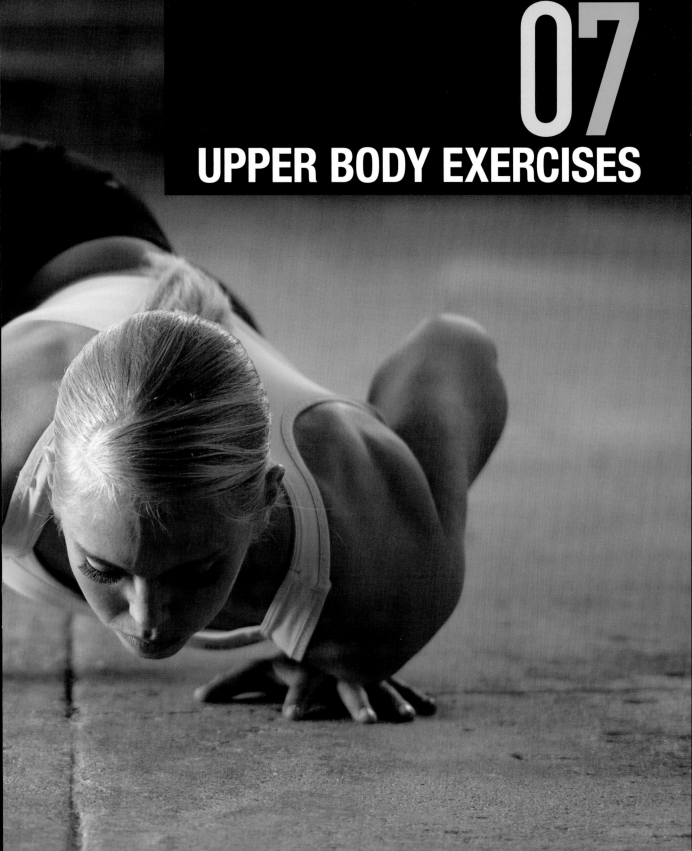

PUSH-UP

The push-up may be the perfect compound exercise. If done correctly, it builds upper body and core strength using the muscles of the chest, back, shoulders, triceps, abs, and even the legs. Keep an eye on your form.

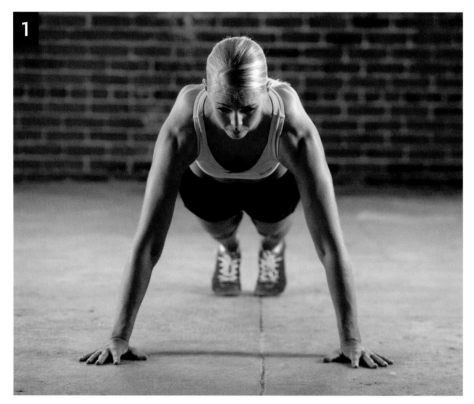

1 Assume a full plank position with your core engaged. Your body should be balanced between your toes and hands, forming a straight line from ankles to head.

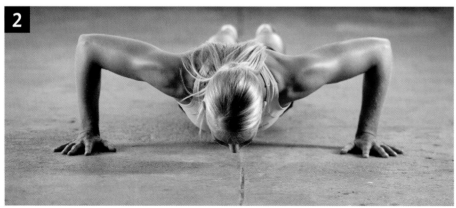

2 Bend your elbows, bringing your chest toward the floor. Once your elbows are slightly beyond 90 degrees, push up through your hands, extending the arms to return to the starting position.

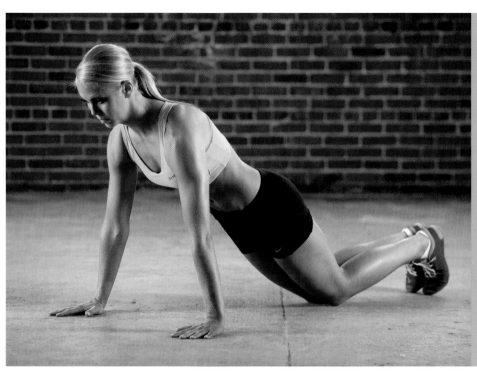

TRAINER TIP
If a full push-up is too challenging, place your knees on the floor for stability and support.

CHALLENGE
There are many push-up variations. Try adjusting the position of your hands to work slightly different muscle groups and make the move more challenging.

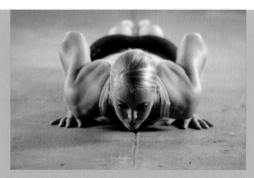

Tricep

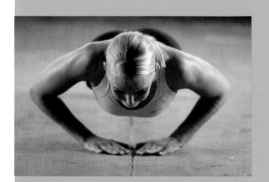

Heart to Hands

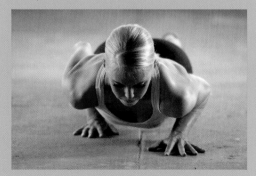

Staggered

CROSS PUSH

Increased core stability makes the cross push a must-do exercise! As your body weight shifts during the crossing phase of the exercise, the muscles used to stabilize your spine (obliques, transverese abdominals, and erector spinae) all engage, helping to build a stronger, tighter tummy.

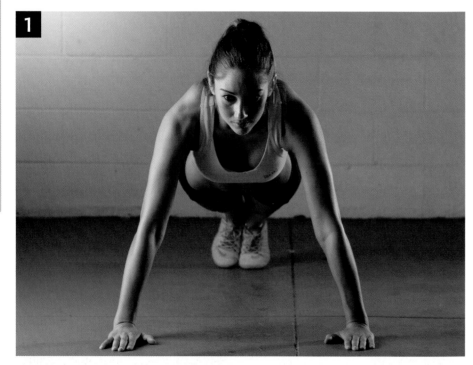

1 Assume a full plank position, with your hands slightly wider than shoulder-width apart and your body forming a straight line from ankles to head. Engage the core.

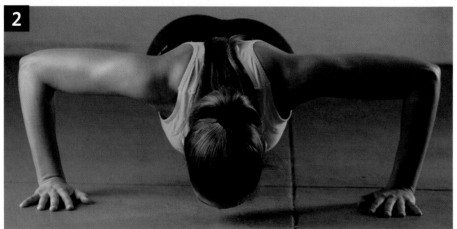

2 Bend your elbows, lowering your chest toward the floor. Once your elbows are slightly beyond 90 degrees, push up through your palms, extending the arms.

3

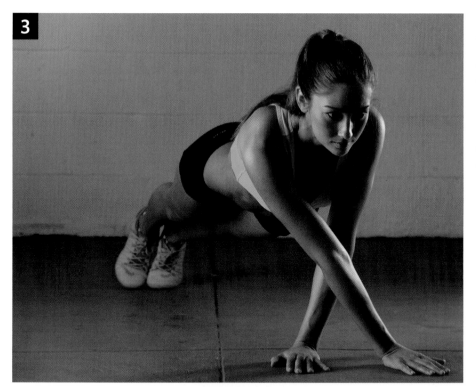

Bring your right hand across the body and briefly place the palm of your right hand on the floor just outside of the left hand. Return the right hand to the starting position. Repeat, alternating the crossing arm.

TRAINER TIP
If a full push-up is too challenging, place your knees on the floor for stability and support

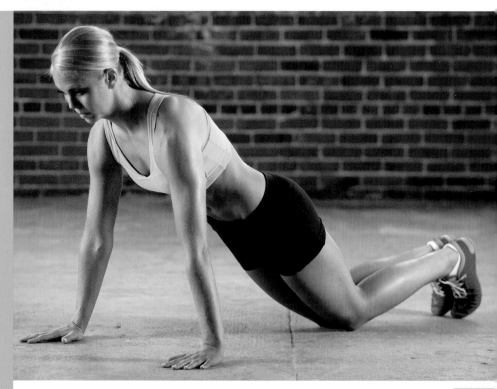

TIGER PUSH-UP

The tiger push-up is one of the most beneficial and comprehensive body weight exercises you can do. This efficient and functional movement engages the shoulders, back, hips, legs, and especially the core. Focus on slow, controlled motion as you perform this exercise.

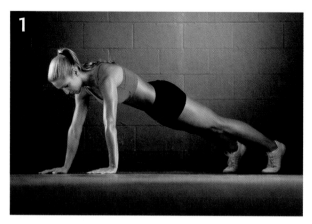

Begin in a standard push-up position, with feet hip-distance apart and hands below shoulders.

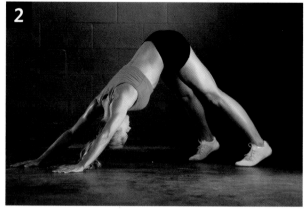

Widen the feet slightly and lift hips into the air, forming an upside-down V-shape. Lengthen the spine and shift weight back into hamstrings and core. Keep your head down.

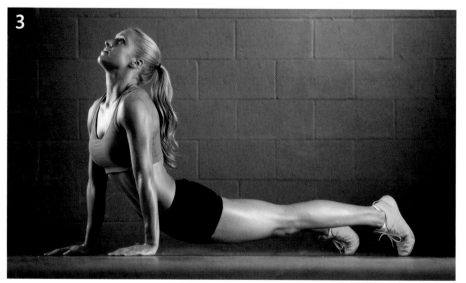

In a controlled diving motion, bring your core down so that your hips move toward the floor as your head and chest lift. (Imagine a golf ball between your hands that you are trying to roll forward with the tip of your nose.)

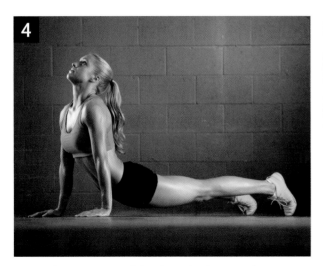

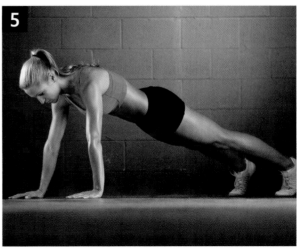

At the deepest point of the dive, slowly extend your body forward so that your back is arched and you are looking up.

While keeping your hips square, lift them up and back to return to the starting position.

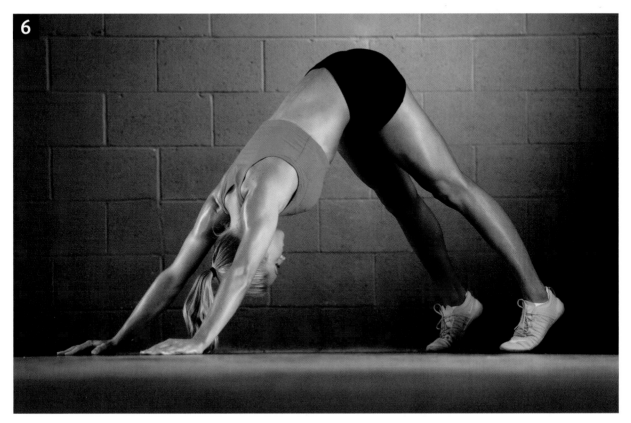

Extend through the spine at the end of the motion as if someone were pulling your hips backward. You will feel this in your hamstrings.

1-2 PUSH

The 1-2 push is an intense, full-body move that will elevate your heart rate while working the muscles in your core, arms, and legs. Complete the move as quickly as you can, but remember that form comes first.

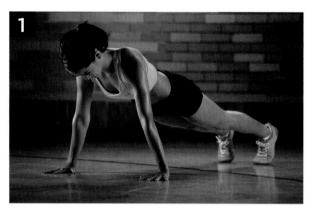

Beginning on all fours, position your hands on the floor slightly wider than your shoulders. Extend your legs and rise up onto your toes, engaging the core and forming a straight line from ankles to head.

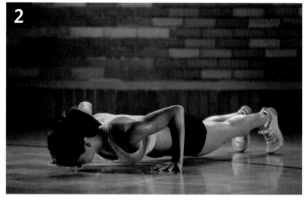

Bend your elbows, bringing the chest toward the floor. When your elbows are bent slightly beyond 90 degrees, push up off the floor and extend the arms.

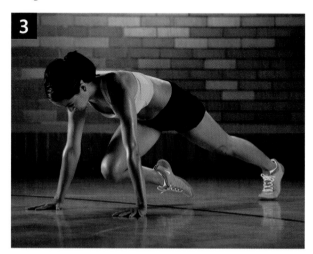

As arms reach full extension, bring your right knee to your chest. Do not lift your hips. Imagine bringing your knee through your elbows.

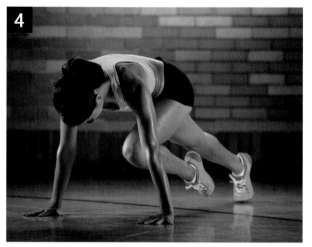

Quickly switch legs, bringing the left knee to the chest. Return to the starting position and repeat.

TRICEP DIP

This targeted exercise is specifically designed to strengthen and define your triceps, the muscles on the underside of your arm between the elbow and the shoulder. If you want to banish wobbly underarms, this is the move for you.

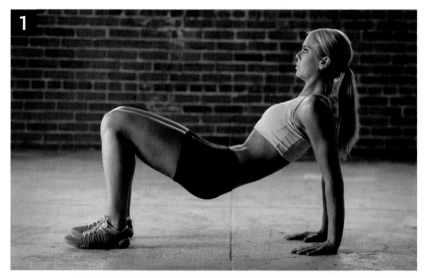

Sit with your feet flat on the floor in front of you and knees slightly bent. Lean back slightly and place your hands on the floor behind your hips, fingers pointing toward your toes. Elevate the hips by engaging the core, hamstrings, and glutes.

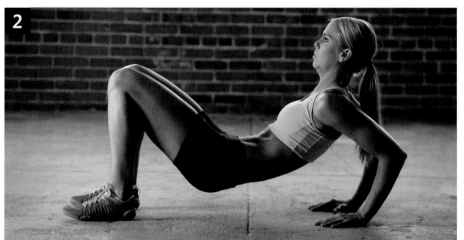

CHALLENGE

For a deeper movement, you can do tricep dips with your hands on a stable, elevated surface, such as a bench.

Bend your elbows, lowering your hips until they're just above the floor. Don't let your elbows flare out. Imagine squeezing your elbows together as you lower your hips. Extend your arms, bringing your hips back up to starting position.

CRAB TOUCH

The crab touch builds on the tricep dip with a coordinated arm and leg movement to further engage your core. Be sure to maintain proper form as you complete the movement. Control is the key to doing this exercise successfully.

1

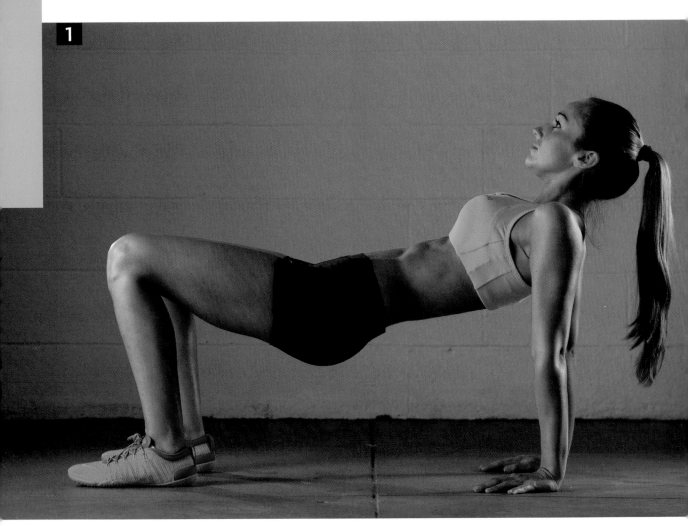

Sit with feet flat on the floor in front of you, back slightly reclined, and hands on the floor just behind your hips with fingers pointing at heels. Raise your hips off the floor, supporting your body weight between the hands and feet. Keep hips elevated and engage the glutes.

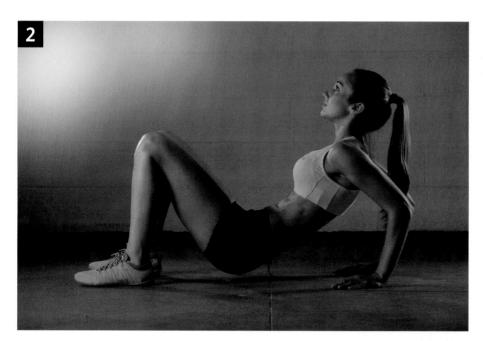

2

Bend your elbows, lowering your hips until they're just above the floor.

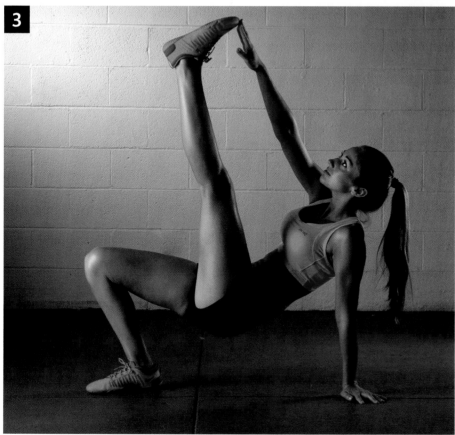

3

Press up through the palms of your hands, extending the arms and driving up through the hips. Raise your left hand and right leg and attempt to touch your toes. Return to the starting position and repeat with the opposite leg.

REACH

The reach is a compound exercise that will target your body's trouble zones while challenging your balance. Pay attention to your form as you complete this exercise.

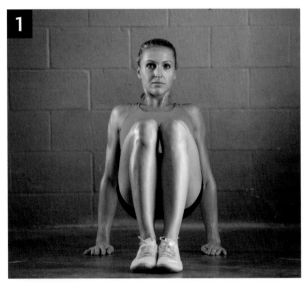

Sit with your feet flat on the floor in front of you, back slightly reclined, and hands on the floor near your hips with fingers pointing at heels. Raise your butt off the floor, supporting your body weight between your hands and feet. Keep hips elevated.

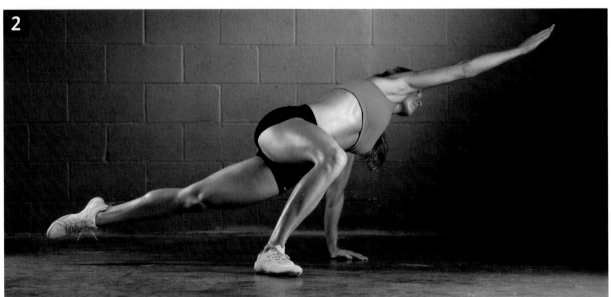

Thread left leg behind right leg as you lift right hand off the floor. Extend both right arm and left leg as far as possible, pulling up through the bottom of the rib cage. Hold for a second.

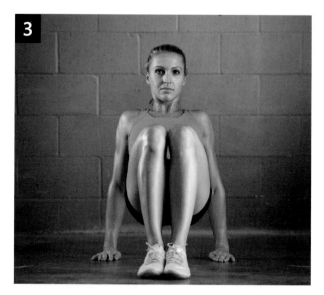

Bring left foot and right hand to the floor, returning to the starting position.

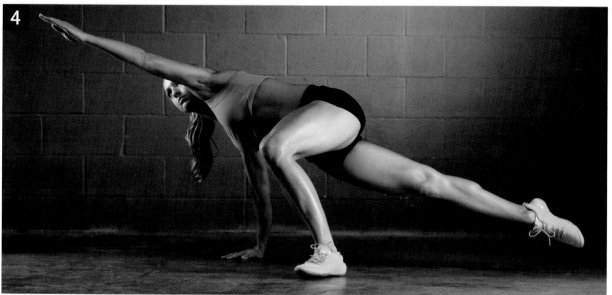

Thread right leg behind left leg as you lift left hand off the floor. Extend right leg and left arm as far as possible and pause for a second. Return to the starting position and repeat, alternating sides. Keep hips elevated, core tight, and glutes engaged.

BALL PRESS

The ball press combines an isolation hold with a press to make your quads, thighs, calves, and butt burn while sculpting your shoulders, back, and arms. Keep your movements quick and explosive while maintaining proper form.

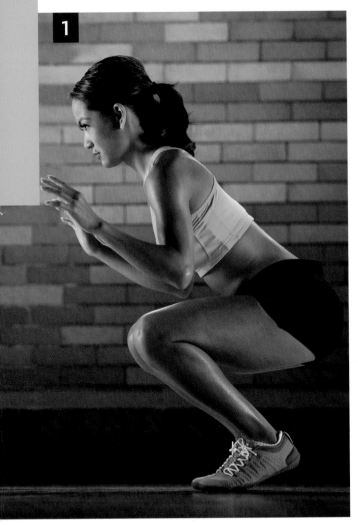

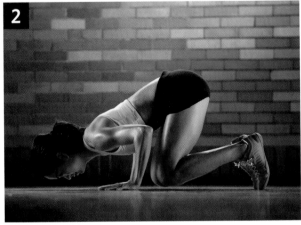

Allow your body to fall forward, catching yourself with your hands and lowering into a mini push-up.

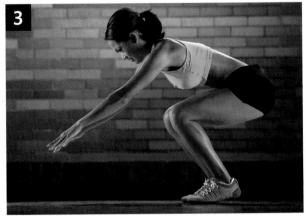

Stand with feet hip-width apart. Rise onto the balls of your feet and lower into a squat position by bending at the hips and knees. Hold your hands in front of your chest with arms bent. This is the "ball" position.

Drive aggressively through the hands to extend the arms and project yourself back onto the balls of your feet, never leaving the "ball" position.

SPHINX

Named after the Egyptian statue, this exercise combines a forearm plank and push-up to work the chest, triceps, back, core, and hips. It is essential to engage your core throughout this exercise for stability and to protect your lower back.

TRAINER TIP
If you find it difficult to extend both arms at the same time, build strength by extending one at a time. Follow a pattern of up, up, down, down (right, left, right, left), switching the lead arm with every rep.

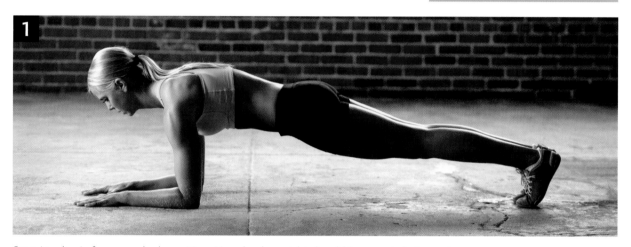

Start in a basic forearm plank position. Your body weight should be evenly balanced between your forearms and toes. Open your hands so that your palms are flat on the floor. Keep your core engaged and body straight.

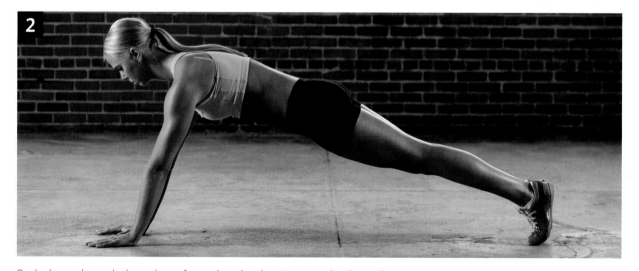

Push down through the palms of your hands, elevating your body until arms are straight. Slowly lower back down into a forearm plank and repeat.

SPIDERMAN

This variation on the push-up is inspired by the agile superhero of the same name. It will increase hip mobility, flexibility, and build core strength.

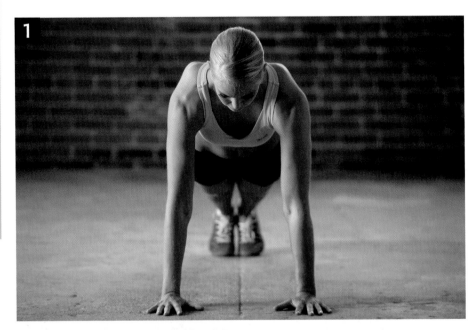

Assume a standard push-up position, with palms just wider than shoulders, arms straight, and body in a straight line balanced between arms and toes.

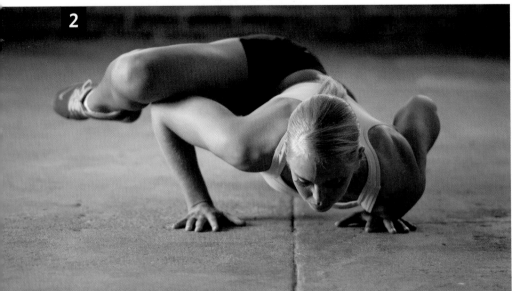

Bend your arms, bringing the chest down as you lift your right foot off the floor. Swing the right leg out sideways, bring your right knee up toward your right shoulder.

Bring your right foot back to the floor and push your body back to the starting position. Repeat, alternating legs.

SHOULDER PRESS JACK

This twist on the classic jumping jack focuses on the latissimus dorsi, or lats, the largest muscles in your back. Concentrate on keeping the lats engaged and use explosive movements to boost your heart rate.

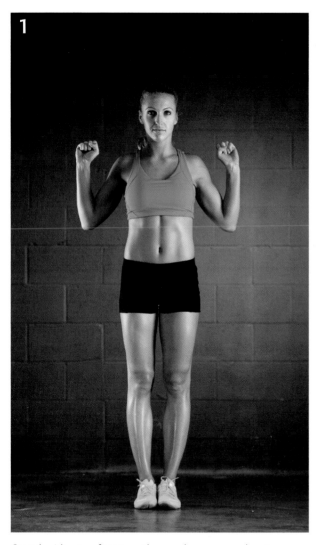

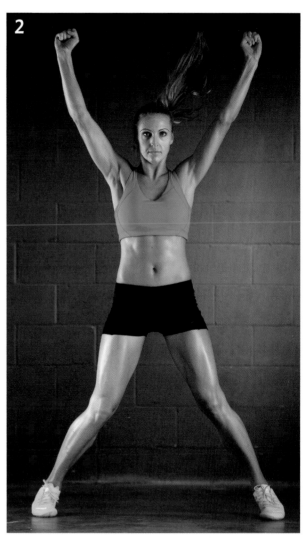

Stand with your feet together and your arms bent, elbows by your sides. Make your hands into fists and concentrate on engaging your lats. Engage the core and soften the knees.

Jump up, opening your feet wider than your shoulders and simultaneously punching your arms toward the roof. Jump again, bringing the feet together as you tuck your elbows back into your sides and concentrate on squeezing and engaging the lats. Repeat.

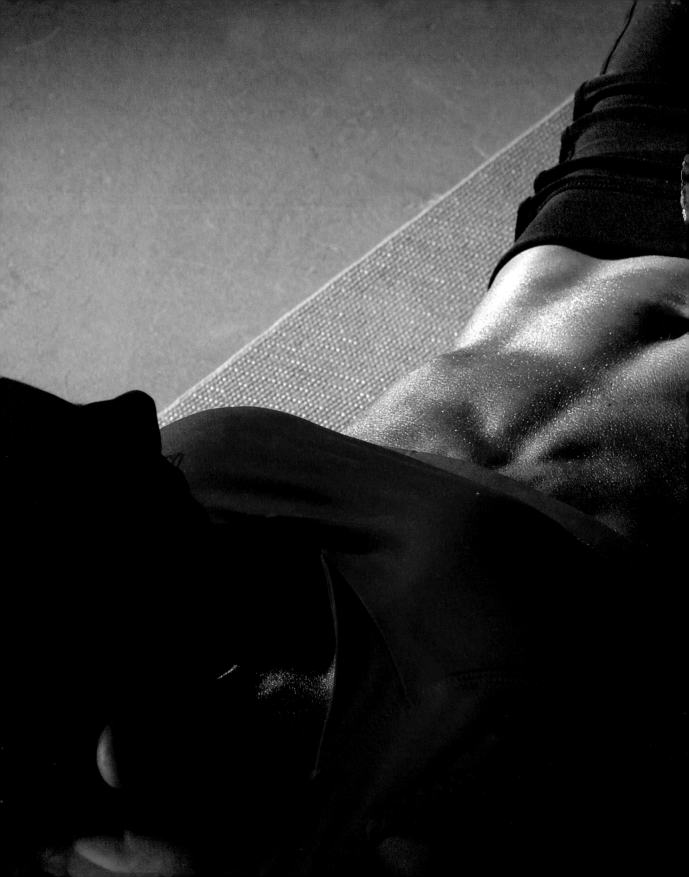

CORE EXERCISES

08

PLANK

This deceptively simple exercise is the secret to rock-hard abs. The plank position engages the transverse abdominals, which aid in stabilization of the spine and pull in the tummy. It helps develop strength in the core, shoulders, and glutes.

CHALLENGE
Super-charge your plank with these modifications.

Lift one leg: Lift one leg and extend it upward. Keep your hips square with the ground and resist the urge to rotate.

Lift one arm: Extend one arm straight out in front of you.

Use a stability ball: Rest your forearms on the ball while keeping your toes on the floor.

Place your forearms on the floor and extend your legs until your body is balanced between your toes and forearms. Your elbows should be directly beneath your shoulders and your body should form a straight line from head to heels. Keep your eyes directly over your fists.

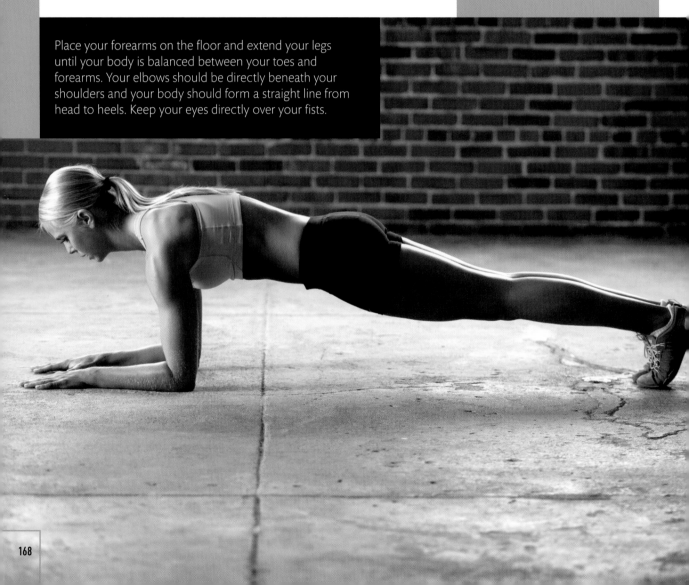

SIDE BEND

If you're looking to get rid of love handles, the side bend will help you do it. This move uses lateral flexion to firm and tighten the internal and external obliques, framing your six-pack abs and creating sleek and sexy definition.

TRAINER TIP
You should not see your arms in your peripheral vision at any time during this exercise. If you see your arms, it is likely you are twisting instead of flexing.

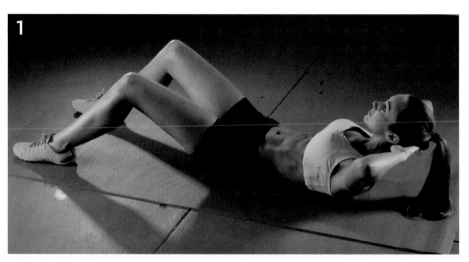

Lay on your back with legs bent and feet resting on the floor. Place your hands behind your head, supporting the neck with fingers interlaced and elbows out wide.

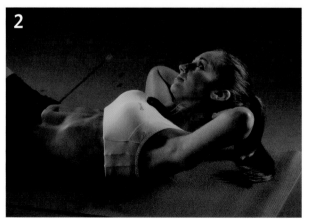

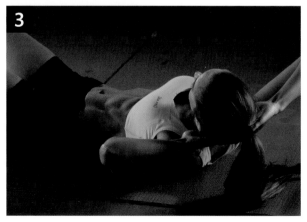

Exhale and pull the right elbow toward the right hip, trying to bend as much as possible.

Inhale and slowly return to the starting position. Repeat on the opposite side.

BICYCLE CRUNCH

The bicycle crunch is an excellent exercise for building core strength and toning the thighs. The movement of your legs mimics the motion of riding a bike.

CHALLENGE
To increase the difficulty of this exercise, elevate the feet. For an even greater challenge, elevate and extend the legs.

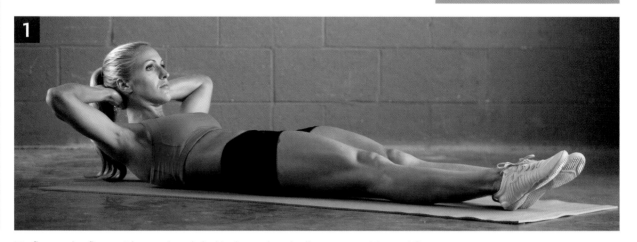

Lie flat on the floor with your hands behind your head, elbows out wide, and fingers interlocked. Pull your shoulder blades off of the floor by activating the abs. Don't pull on your neck.

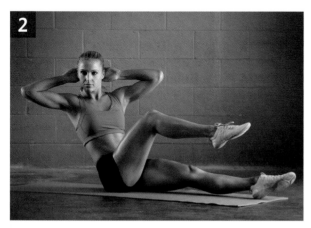

Bring your right knee toward your chest until it is bent at 90 degrees. Simultaneously rotate your core to pull your left shoulder toward the right knee.

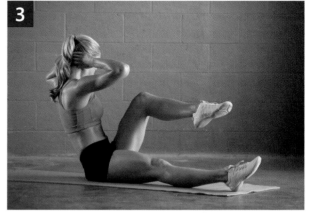

Switch sides, extending the right leg and simultaneously pulling the left knee toward your chest. Rotate your core and pull your right shoulder toward the left knee. Repeat, alternating sides.

RUSSIAN TWIST

This classic ab exercise targets the obliques, but your back muscles will also be engaged to stabilize and support your spine.

CAUTION
Do not do this exercise if you have lower back pain or injury. Substitute the bicycle crunch instead.

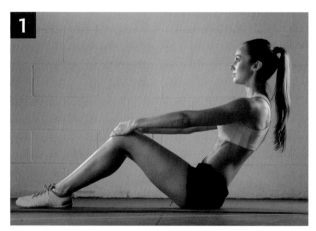

Sit on the ground with heels on the floor, feet approximately one foot in front of you. Hold onto your knees and straighten your arms as you lean back without rounding your spine. This is the perfect position for your spine; don't let it curve during the exercise.

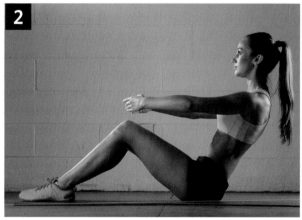

Lift arms from knees and extend in front of rib cage. Arms should remain slightly rounded as if holding a beach ball to your chest.

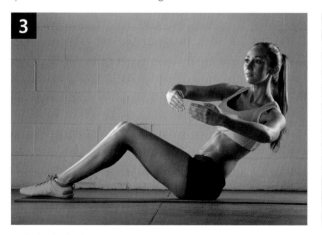

Pull the belly button to the spine and rotate to the left. This is a small controlled motion; do not swing your arms. If you feel pain in your lower back, reduce the amount of twist.

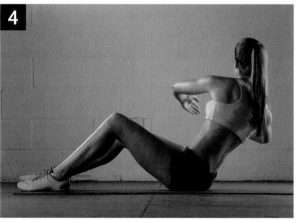

Inhale to center and rotate to the right. Repeat, keeping your abs engaged and spine straight.

PIKE

The pike, or leg raise, is the one ab exercise we always come back to in the gym. Pikes are a simple yet highly effective way to target your lower abs and hip flexors.

CAUTION

If your back arches as the legs lower, you are taking your legs too low. The weight and leverage of the legs is too much for your core to control. Adjust the angle of the legs accordingly to keep the work in the abs and hip flexors.

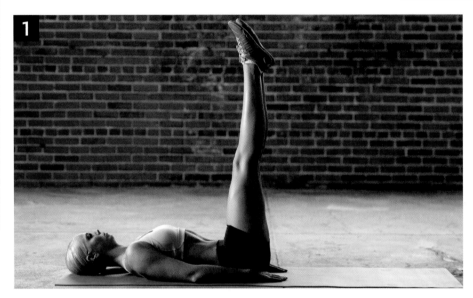

Lie on your back and place your hands under your butt with palms facing down. Squeeze your legs together and slowly raise them until they are perpendicular to the floor, keeping them as straight as possible. Hold the contraction for one second.

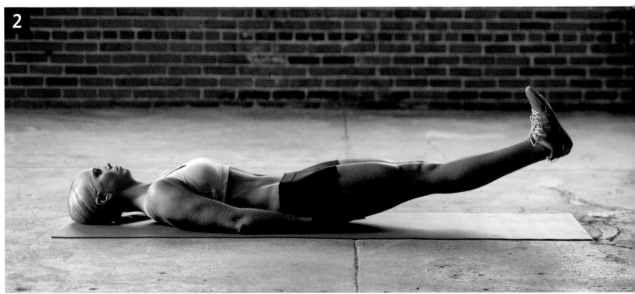

Maintaining straight legs, slowly lower your feet to within an inch of the floor.

IN-AND-OUT ABS

In-and-out abs combines the core work of the classic plank with a dynamic tuck that challenges the thighs and hips and engages stabilizing muscles.

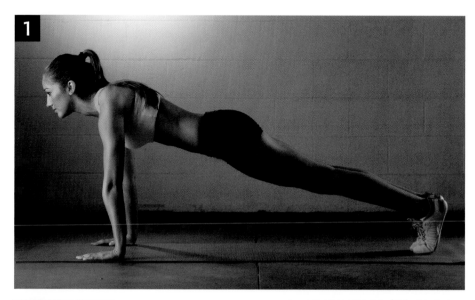

Position your hands on the floor, slightly wider than shoulder-width apart. Rise up onto your toes and engage the core to form a straight line from ankles to head. Squeeze the glutes to support your lower back.

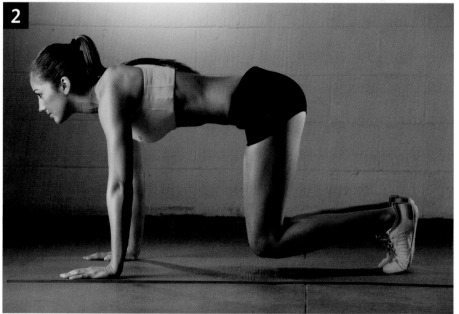

Jump in, tucking both knees under your body and landing on the toes with legs bent at 90 degrees. Do not bring your knees past your hips.

Jump back to the starting position, engaging the core for stability.

ROW BOAT

Challenge your balance and torch your hip flexors, abs, and thighs with this dynamic movement inspired by the movement of rowers.

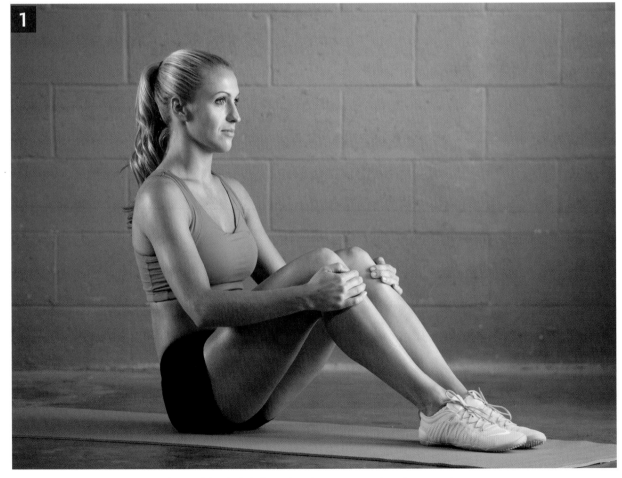

Sit on the floor with your feet flat and back slightly reclined. Wrap your hands around your shins.

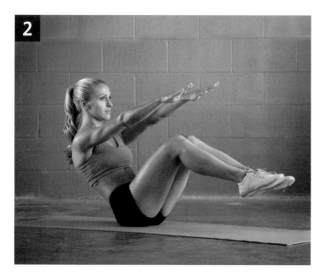

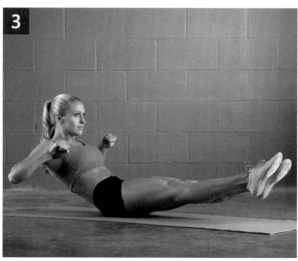

Elevate your feet and find your balance by engaging your core. Then extend your arms out straight in front of you. Pull your belly button inward. Keep the spine straight.

Pull your elbows back in a rowing motion as you simultaneously extend your legs. Squeeze your shoulder blades and inner thighs.

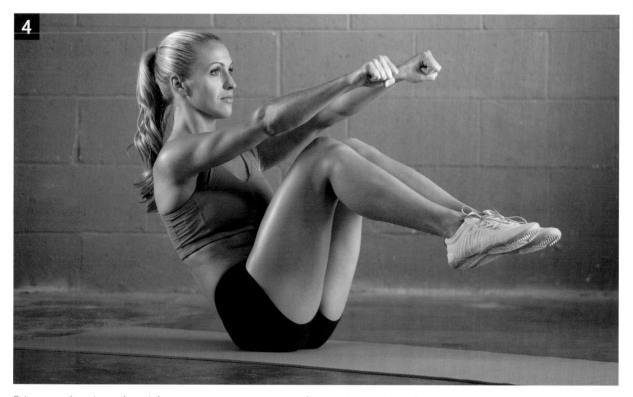

Bring your legs in and straighten your arms to return to the starting position. Repeat without resting feet on the floor.

SIDE PLANK

The side plank will tighten and shrink your waistline by working the underlying abdominal muscles (obliques and transverse abs).

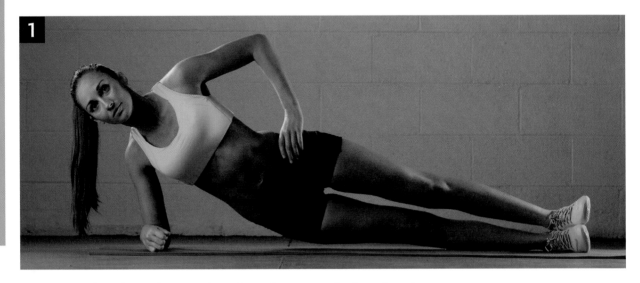

Lie on your side with your legs straight and your forearm on the floor. Rest the non-working arm on your hip or behind your head.

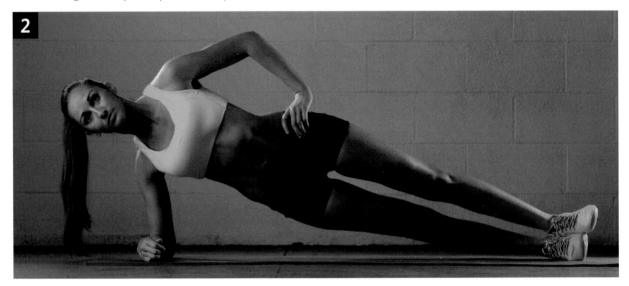

Lift up at the hips, creating a straight line from head to heels. Hold the position.

CHALLENGE

Super-charge your side planks by lifting and lowering your hips, or by incorporating these variations.

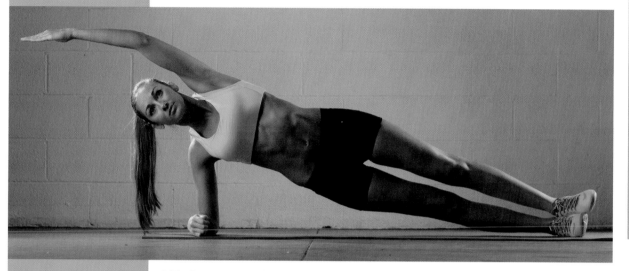

Lift the arm overhead: This lengthens your body and challenges your stabilizing muscles.

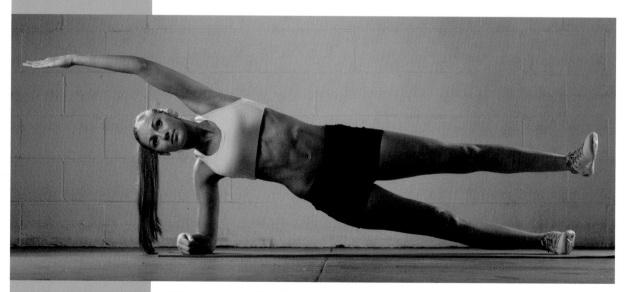

Lift the top leg: This increases the load on both your core and the stabilizing leg, challenging both strength and balance.

PLANK PUNCH

The classic plank is an exceptional exercise for the core and for developing shoulder stability. Adding a controlled punching movement increases core stabilization as you are forced to resist rotation of the hips and shoulders.

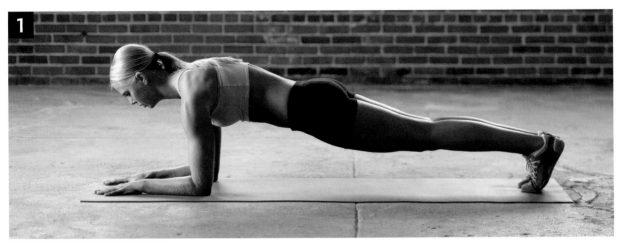

Place your forearms on the floor and extend your legs until your body is balanced between your toes and forearms. Your elbows should be directly beneath your shoulders and your body should form a straight line from head to heels.

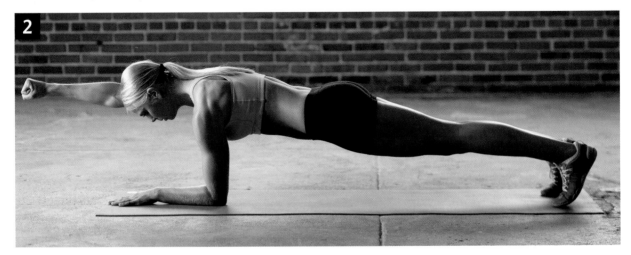

Raise one arm and punch forward. Extend your arm straight out as you punch at shoulder height, parallel to the floor. Return to the starting position and repeat with the opposite arm.

PLANK ROTATION

Plank rotations are a fun alternative to the traditional side plank. Rotating the body through multiple planes of motion challenges your balance and coordination and will tone the obliques, back, hips, thighs, and shoulders.

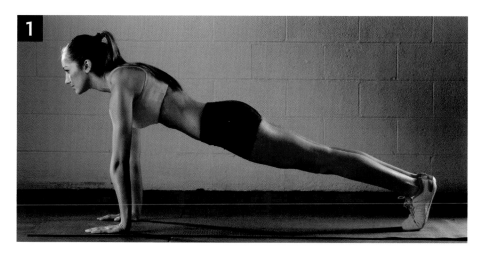

Begin in a full push-up position, with wrists under shoulders, core engaged, and legs extended.

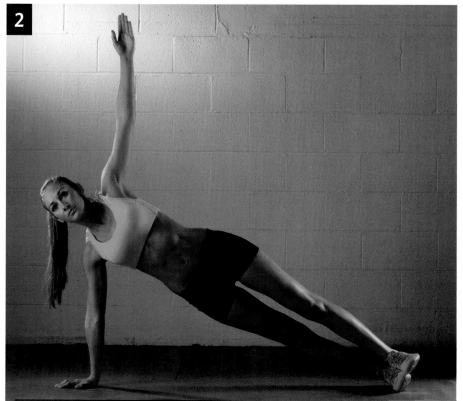

Raise your left arm toward the ceiling as you slowly rotate your body to the left. Lift from the bottom of the rib cage, opening the chest. Return to the starting position and repeat on the opposite side.

UP, UP, DOWN, DOWN

This exercise takes the six-pack abs (rectus abdominus) through three types of muscle contraction: isolation during the pause, concentric as you sit up, and eccentric as you lower back down. It's an incredible way to tone, tighten, and strengthen your core.

1

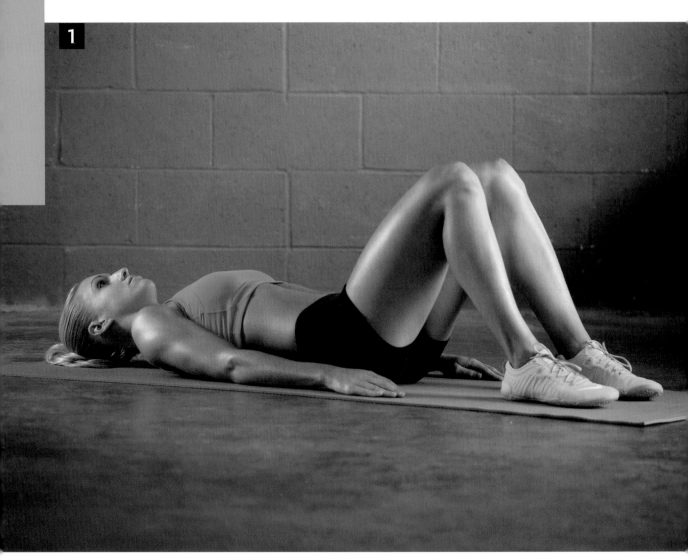

Lie on your back with your legs bent and feet flat on the floor. Extend your arms by your sides.

TRAINER TIP

Remember that this is not a sit-up. Move slowly and exaggerate the pauses.

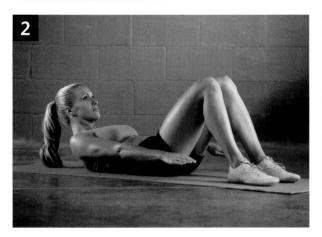

Exhale and lift your chest up so just your shoulder blades are off the floor. Focus on engaging the top two upper abdominal muscles. Pause.

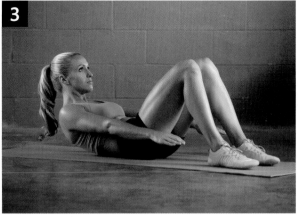

Continue to exhale and lift up further, pulling the belly button to the spine and mentally engaging the remaining abdominals. Reach your fingertips just past your knees. Pause.

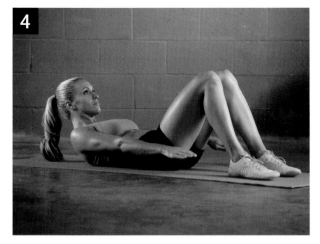

Inhale as you slowly begin to curl back down. Pause with the shoulder blades just lifted off the floor.

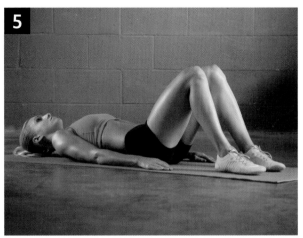

Lower your body completely, returning to the starting position. Repeat with control, exaggerating the pauses.

DIAGONAL PIKE

Leg raises are a simple yet highly effective way to target your lower abs and hip flexors. The addition of the diagonal movement increases the workload of your obliques.

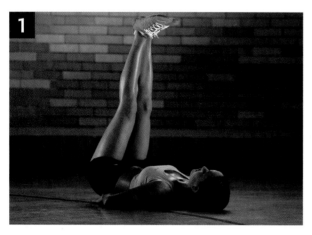

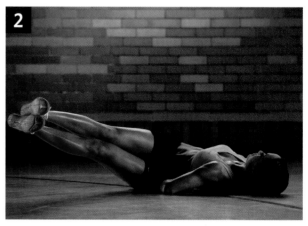

Lie on your back with your hands under your butt, palms facing down. Keep your legs as straight as possible and squeeze them together. Raise the legs until they are perpendicular to the floor.

Lower your legs to the left at a 45-degree angle, until feet are just above the floor. Pause before returning to the starting position.

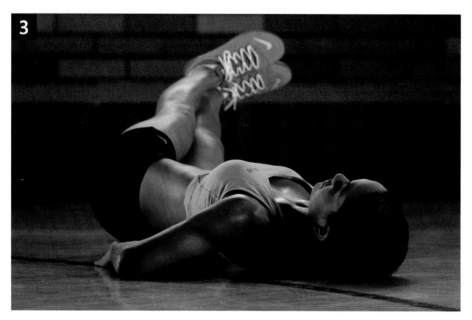

Lower your legs to the right at a 45-degree angle, until feet are just above the floor. Pause before returning to the starting position and repeat.

V-UP

The V-up takes its name from the shape your body forms during the exercise. This advanced ab exercise engages the six-pack abdominal muscles, the erector muscles of the spine, and the hip flexors. V-ups require great coordination as well as balance.

1

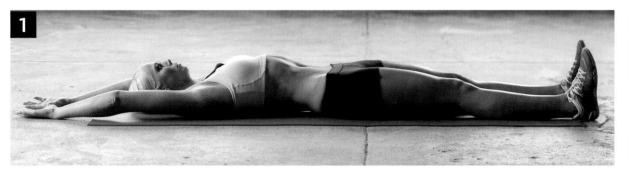

Lie on your back with arms and legs straight. Extend your arms above your head. Keep your pelvis flat and a natural arch to your back.

2

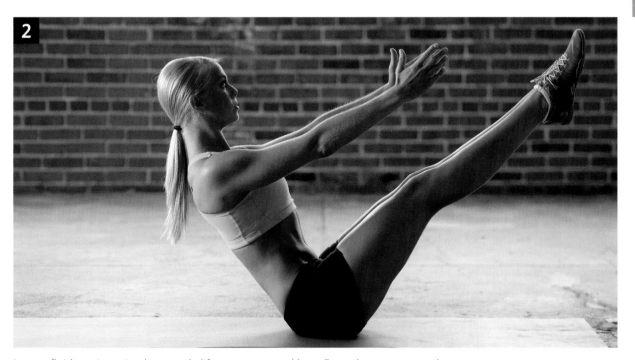

In one fluid motion, simultaneously lift your torso and legs. Extend your arms so they are parallel to the legs and keep your head in line with your body. Control the body back to the starting position and repeat.

DOUBLE CROSS REACH

The double cross reach will test your balance and coordination while working your abs, back, thighs, and hip flexors.

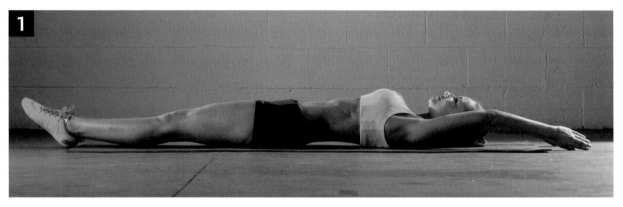

Lie on your back with legs straight and arms extended above your head. Keep your pelvis flat and a natural arch to your back.

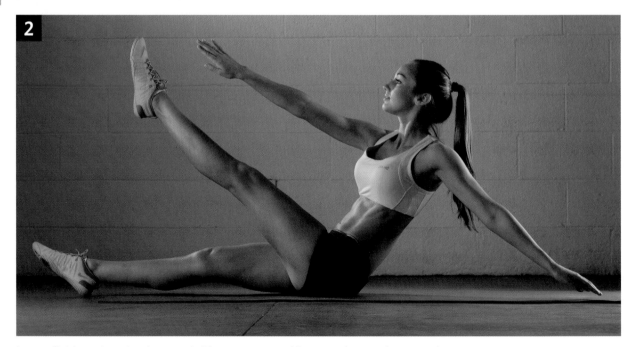

In one fluid motion, simultaneously lift your torso and legs, reaching with your right hand across the body to touch the toes of your left foot. Do not allow the lower back to collapse.

CAUTION
This advanced exercise can stress the lower back. If you have low back pain or injury, substitute the bicycle crunch instead.

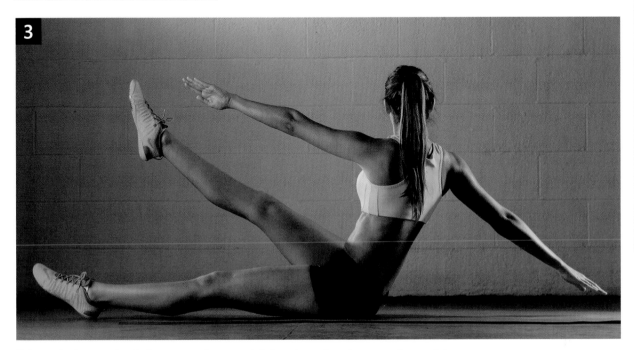

Scissor the legs and switch arms so that your left hand touches the toes of your right foot. Keep your torso tall.

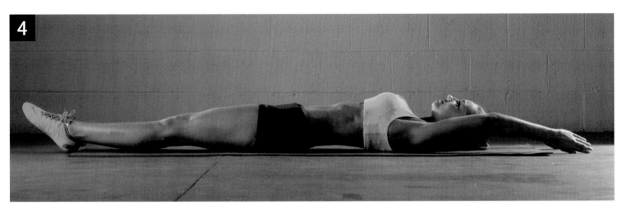

Slowly lower back to the starting position and repeat, this time beginning by touching the left hand to the toes of the right foot.

OPEN-AND-CLOSE PIKE

Open-and-close pikes add a little fun to the traditional leg raise. In addition to challenging your stabilizing core muscles, opening and closing the legs at the top of the movement helps tone the inner and outer thighs, hips, and glutes.

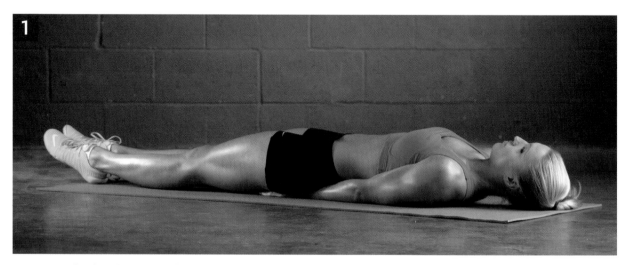

Lie on your back with your hands under your butt, palms facing down. Keep your legs as straight as possible and squeeze them together.

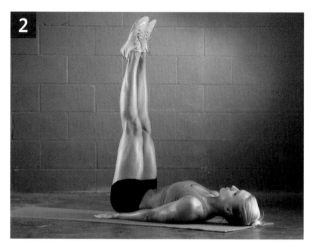

Slowly raise your legs until they are perpendicular to the floor.

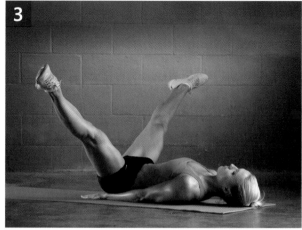

Open your legs as wide as possible.

CAUTION
If your back arches as the legs lower, you are taking your legs too low. Lift your legs to keep the work in the abs and hip flexors.

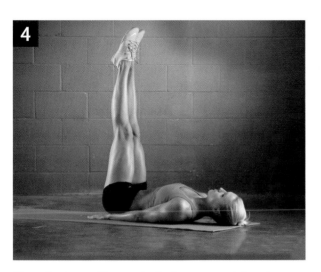

Close the legs with a controlled movement, keeping them straight and perpendicular to the floor.

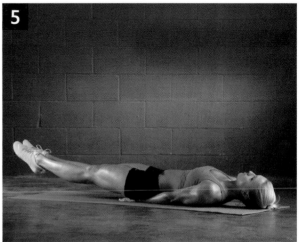

Slowly lower the feet until they are just above the floor.

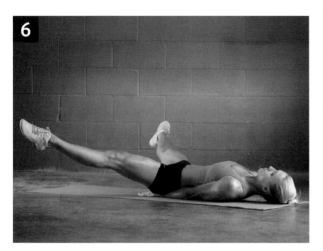

Keeping your feet just above the floor, open your legs as wide as possible with a slow, controlled movement.

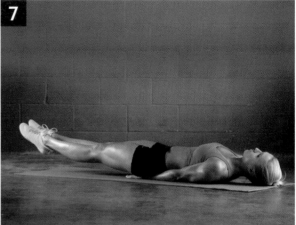

Close the legs and begin the sequence again by raising your legs until they are perpendicular to the floor. Do not allow your feet to touch the floor.

SPRINTER SIT-UP

This is no ordinary sit-up. The alternating movements of the arms and legs force your stabilizing core muscles to work, while aggressively driving the knees works the hip flexors.

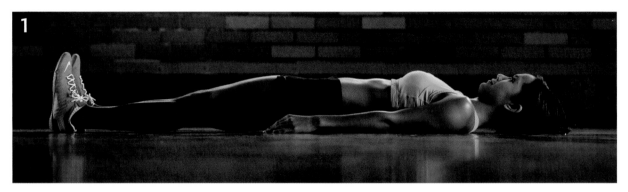

Lie on your back with your arms at your sides and legs extended.

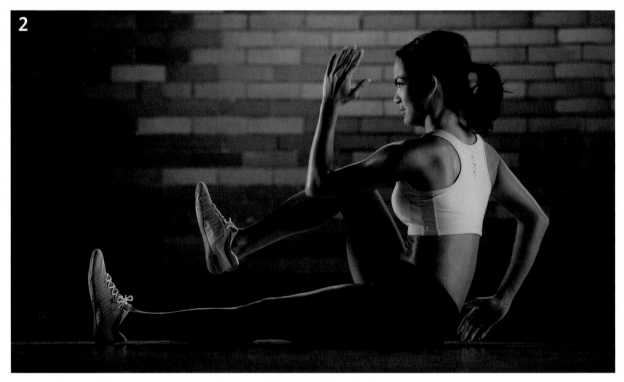

Sit up with an explosive movement, simultaneously bringing the right knee to your chest and swinging the left arm forward as if running.

CAUTION
Do not rotate your torso while swinging your arms. Keep your hips and shoulders facing forward.

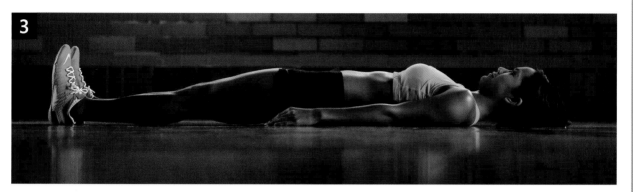

Fully extend the right leg and return the left arm to the starting position.

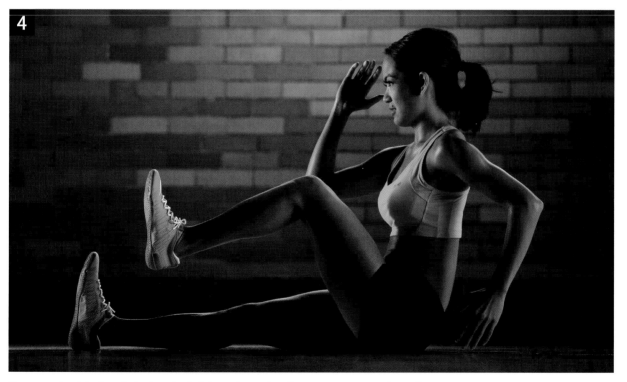

Sit up again, this time bringing the left knee in to the chest as you swing the right arm forward. Repeat, alternating arm and leg movements as though sprinting.

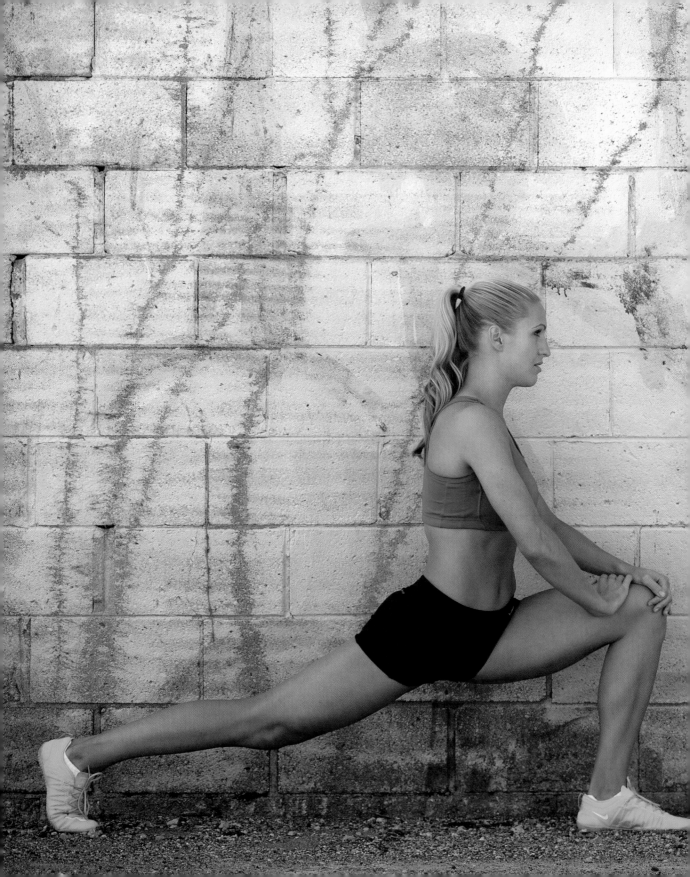

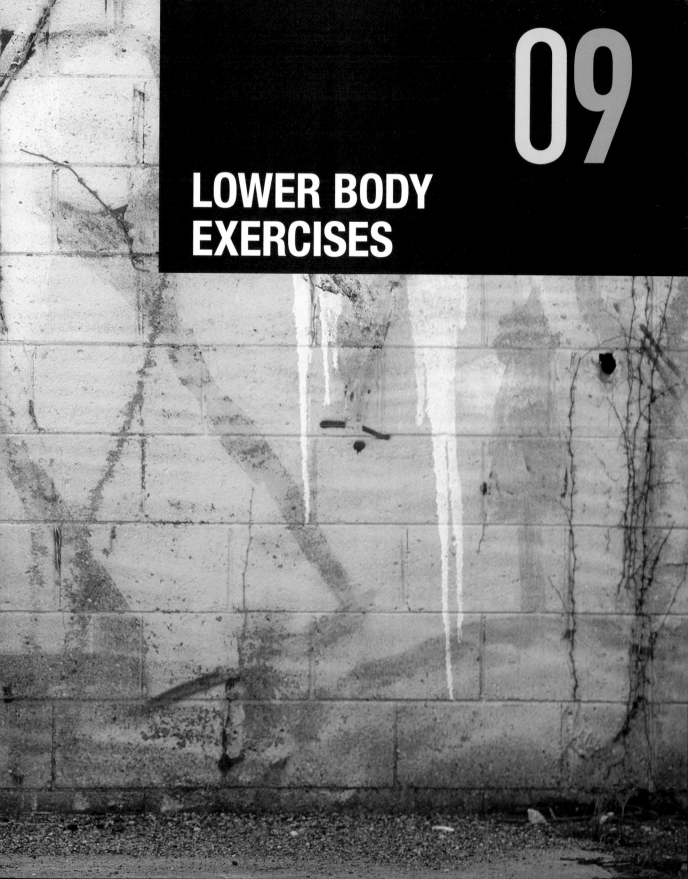

09

LOWER BODY EXERCISES

SQUAT JUMP

A metabolic-boosting super exercise, the squat jump demands every ounce of energy and coordination while making the large muscles of the lower body scream.

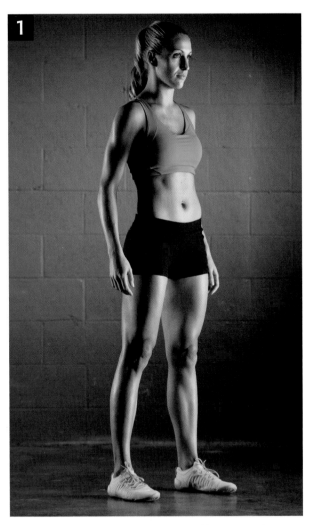

Stand tall with your feet shoulder-width apart and your toes pointing forward.

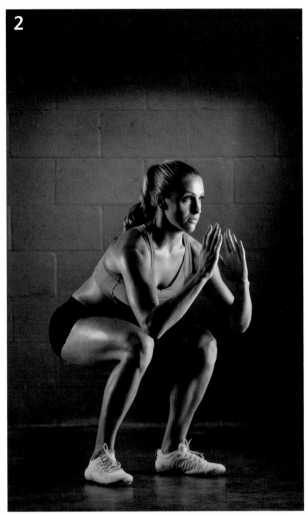

With your weight in your heels, inhale as you bend at the knee and lower your body into a squat. Your torso should be tall and your core engaged.

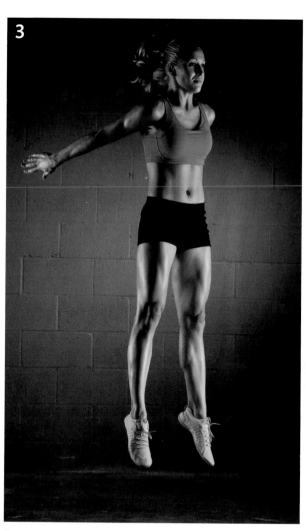

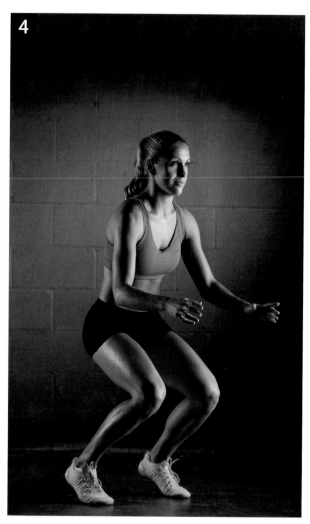

Engage your core and exhale as you jump up, pushing through the heels. Swing your arms as you jump to generate momentum.

Land as softly and silently as possible, bending at the ankles, knees, and hips to decelerate the body.

SQUAT HOLD

A simple variation on the traditional squat, the squat hold is used to build isometric strength but will also tone your thighs, hips, and butt. Be prepared to feel the burn.

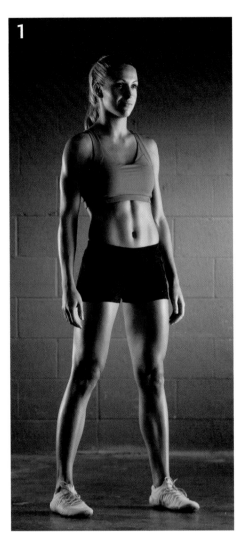

Stand tall, feet shoulder width and toes pointing forward.

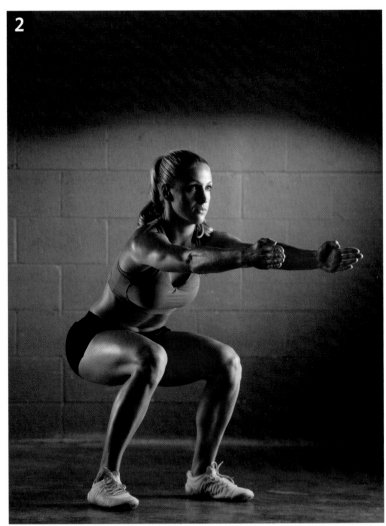

With your weight in your heels, inhale as you bend at the knee, lowering your body until the thighs are parallel to the floor. Extend your arms for balance and hold.

LATERAL LUNGE

Lateral lunges increase dynamic balance, strengthening and toning the glutes, hamstrings, and thighs in the process.

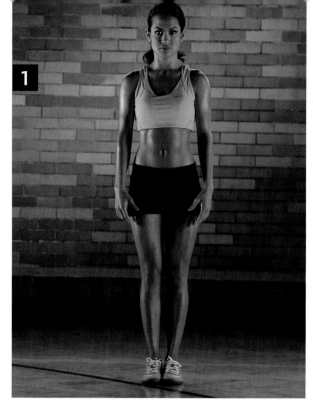

Stand tall with arms at your sides and toes pointing forward.

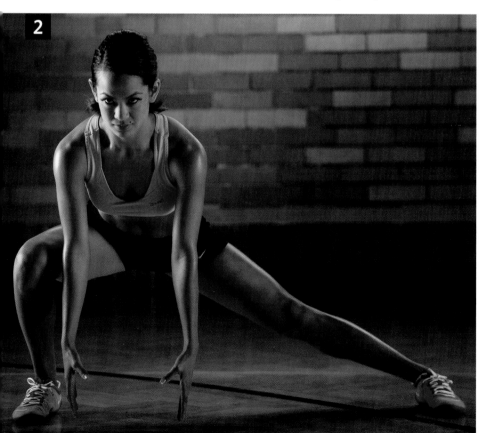

Step out to the side (laterally) away from the body. Remain tall and keep your weight in your heels as you push back your hips, lowering your body until the thigh is parallel to the floor.

Push back off of the bent leg, extending hips and knee to return to your starting position.

4 CALF RAISES + 4 TAPS

This exercise combination is inspired by ballet movements. It's designed to tone and strengthen your calves while raising your heart rate and strengthening your quads with plyometric motion.

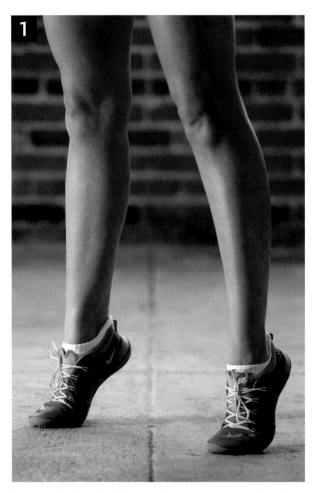

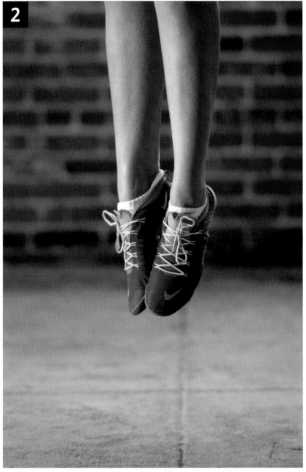

Stand with feet shoulder-width apart. Raise your heels until you are balancing on the balls of your feet. Slowly lower until your heels return to the floor. Repeat four times. Lift as high as possible on each calf raise.

Bend slightly at the knees and in one fluid yet dynamic motion, explode off the floor and lightly tap the insteps of your feet together. Land softly, bending at the hips, knees, and ankles. Repeat four times.

SKATER JUMP

This exercise mimics the movement of a speed skater moving across the ice. Skater jumps will strengthen your legs, improve balance and coordination, and raise your heart rate.

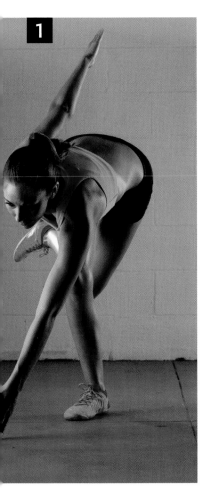

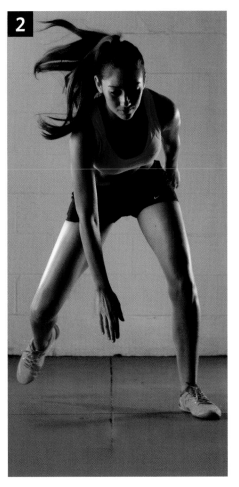

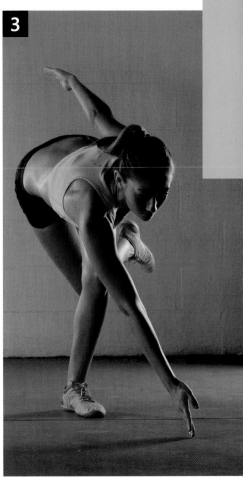

Stand with your weight on your right foot and a soft bend in the knee. Lift your left leg and cross it behind the right leg as you bring your left hand to the floor.

Bound to the left by pushing off of your right foot. Bring your right arm forward and your left arm back as you jump.

Land on your left foot and bring the right foot behind your left, touching your right hand to the floor. Repeat. You should be able to move from side to side in one fluid movement.

SQUAT

The squat is a compound, full-body exercise that primarily engages the muscles of the thighs, hips, and glutes. It also helps to develop core strength by engaging the lower back and abdominals.

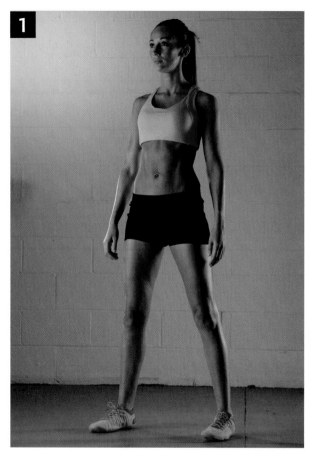

Stand tall, with your feet shoulder-width apart and toes pointing forward.

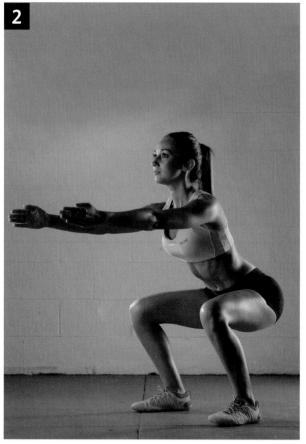

Inhale as you bend at the knees, lowering your body as if about to sit in a chair. At the bottom of the movement, your knees should be at a 90-degree angle and your thighs parallel to the ground. Keep your knees over your ankles and your torso tall.

SKI JUMP

This exercise is inspired by the movement of downhill skiing. It will condition the calves, quads, and glutes while kicking up your heart rate and challenging your balance, coordination, and core stabilization.

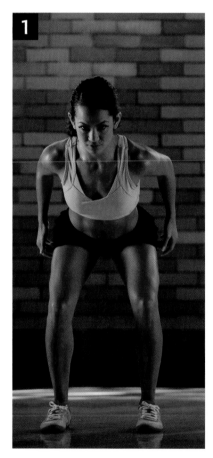

1

Stand tall with your toes pointing forward and your weight in your heels. Inhale as you bend at the knees, lowering into a half squat.

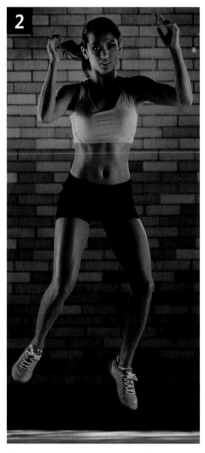

2

Engage your core and exhale as you jump to one side with both feet, maintaining the distance between them. Keep your hips and shoulders facing forward, and bend your arms as though holding ski poles.

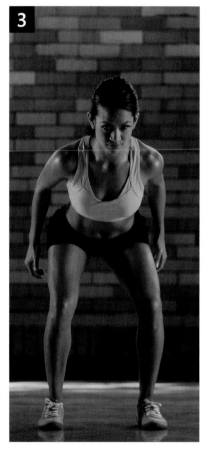

3

Land as softly and silently as possible, bending at the ankles, knees, and hips to decelerate the body back to the half-squat position.

SQUAT PEDAL

This exercise combines squat jumps with jumping lunges to burn more calories than any other bodyweight resistance exercise. This metabolic booster simultaneously activates the thighs, hamstrings, glutes, and core. Keep your movements explosive, but maintain proper form.

TRAINER TIP
If jumping is too strenuous, you can alternate bodyweight squats and reverse lunges.

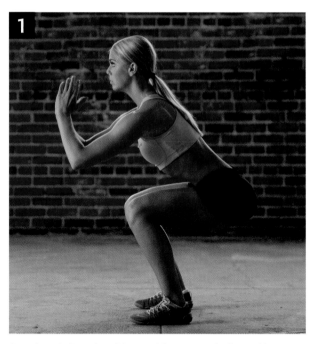

Stand with feet shoulder-width apart. Inhale and lower into a squat.

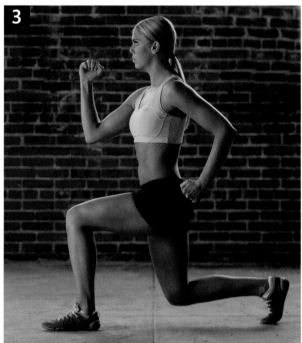

Engage your core and exhale as you jump up. While in the air, scissor-switch your feet.

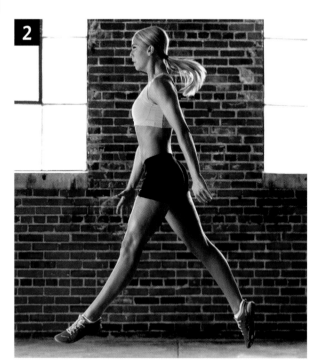

Land with your left foot forward and sink into a lunge.

4

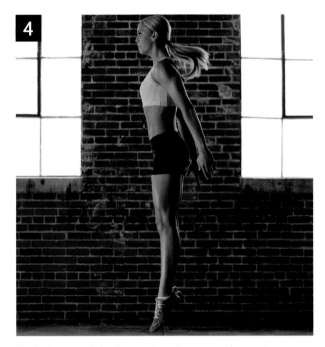

Explode out of the lunge, jumping up and opening your feet laterally, ready to land in the squat position.

5

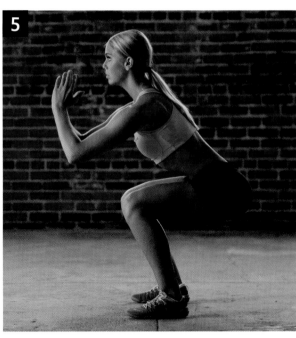

Engage the core and use your ankles, knees, and hips to decelerate your body, landing in a deep squat position.

6

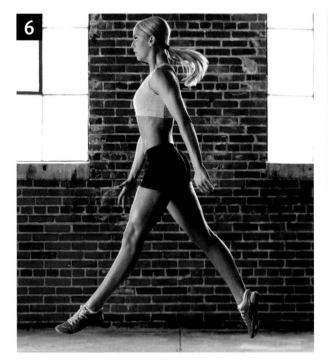

Accelerate through the balls of the feet, jumping with enough force to scissor-switch your feet.

7

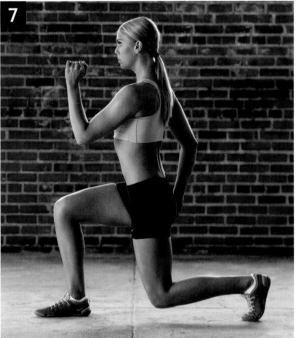

Land with your right foot forward and lower into a lunge. Repeat alternating the front leg on each lunge.

SKI SQUAT

The ski squat is an intense cardio move that builds on the benefits of the traditional squat jump to tone the glutes, thighs, and hamstrings.

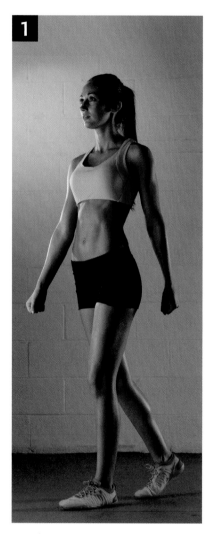

1

Stand in a staggered stance, left foot in front of the right.

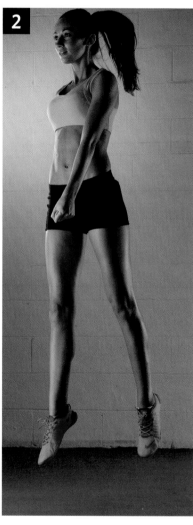

2

Jump with enough force to propel both feet from the floor. While in the air, scissor-switch the feet.

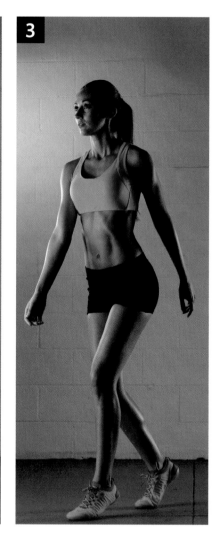

3

Land softly with left foot in front.

TRAINER TIP
Find a cadence with this exercise: left, right, squat; right, left, squat. You should be able to hear a rhythm to your footfalls as you go through the movement.

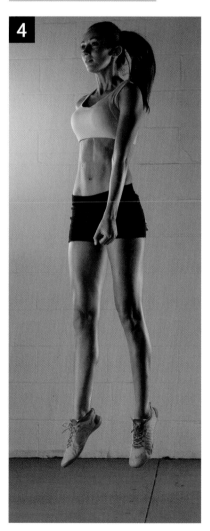

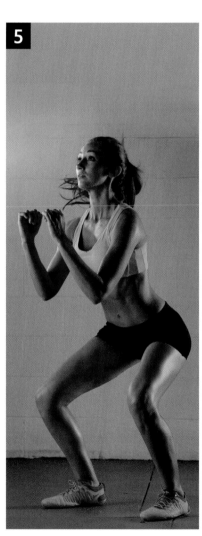

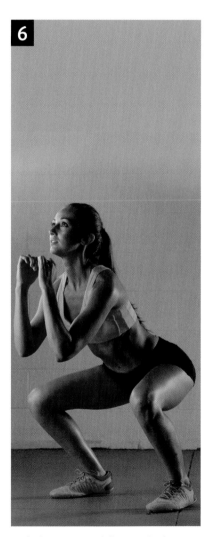

Jump once more, this time opening the feet to hip-width apart and prepare to land in a squat.

Land with a slight bend in the ankles, hips, and knees to decelerate the body. Keep your torso tall and core engaged.

Sink down into a full squat before exploding upward, jumping and switching the feet to land with the right foot in front of the left.

IN AND OUTS

This plyometric squat engages the thighs, glutes, and hamstrings. It will challenge your balance and coordination, activate the core, and tone the lower body.

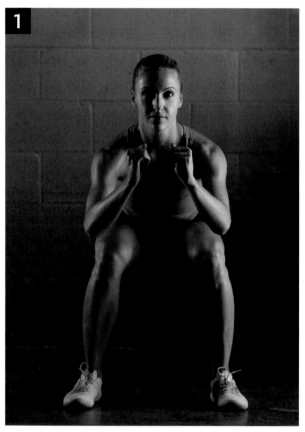

With your weight in your heels, inhale as you bend at the hips and knees, lowering into a squat. Try to bring your thighs parallel to the floor.

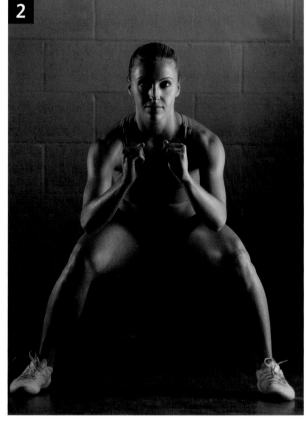

Make the smallest of jumps and open your feet laterally, landing with feet wider than your shoulders. Repeat, staying as low as possible in your squat position and jumping out.

T-STAND

Lengthen the hamstrings and challenge your balance in this yoga-inspired, functional exercise. While it may seem simple, it will make your hamstrings burn.

TRAINER TIP
If balancing is a challenge, allow your arms to drop and your fingertips to touch the floor.

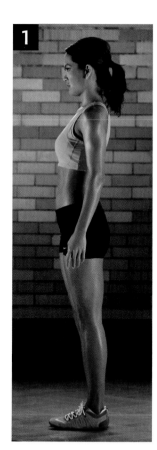

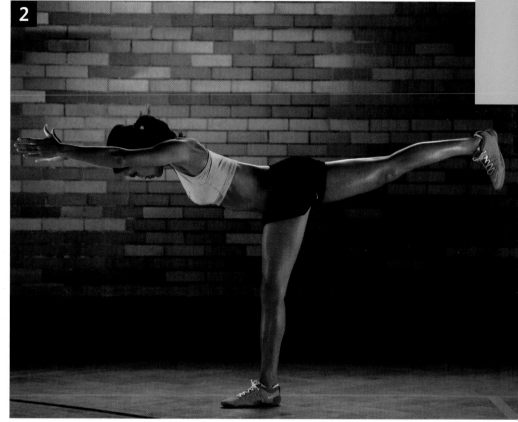

Stand with feet together and arms at your sides.

Inhale and slowly bend from the hips, lowering the torso and extending the arms. As you fold forward, raise one leg until torso, arms, and leg are parallel to the floor. Exhale as you lift the torso and lower the leg in one fluid motion. Repeat with the opposite leg.

JUMP LUNGE

Jump lunges will quickly get your legs burning and your heart rate skyrocketing. This quad-killing exercise requires balance and coordination. Make sure you're maintaining proper form throughout the movement.

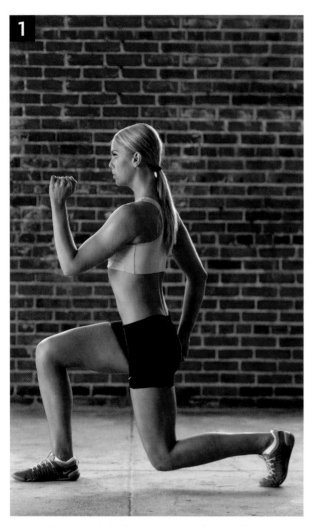

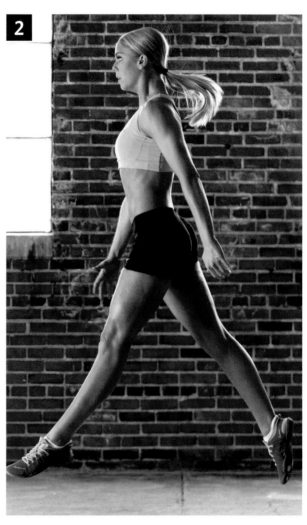

Stand with your right foot in front of the left. Keep your torso as tall as possible as you bend both legs to sink into a lunge position. Don't allow the front knee to go past your toes.

Jump up with enough force to propel both feet from the floor. While in the air, scissor-switch your feet.

CAUTION

Pay particular attention to the impact imposed during the landing. Attempt to land as softly as possible so that the force of the deceleration is distributed between the knee, hip, and ankle joints.

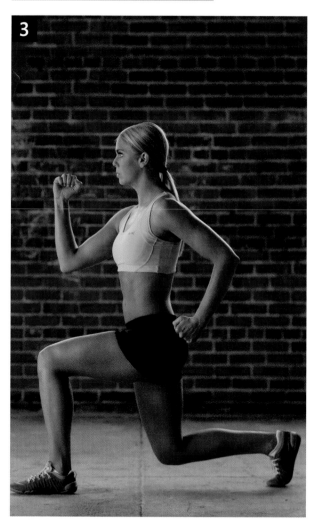

Land softly in a lunge position with the left foot in front.

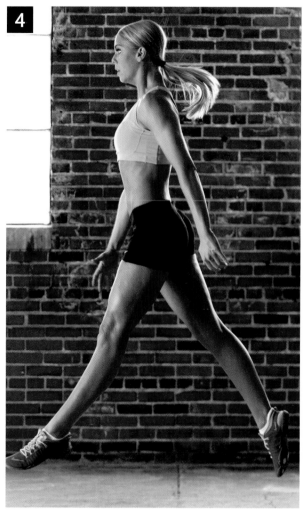

Jump up again, and scissor-switch your feet to land softly in a lunge position with the right leg in front.

UP DOWN

This exercise makes the simple movement of getting up off the floor fun and challenging. Build core stability and strengthen your glutes, thighs, and hamstrings as you move up and then back down.

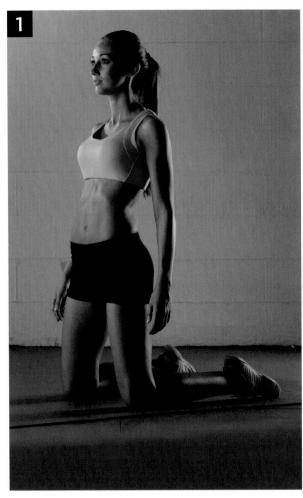

Begin in a kneeling position. Keep your torso tall, with your head up, shoulders back, and core engaged. If kneeling is uncomfortable, place a rolled towel under your knees.

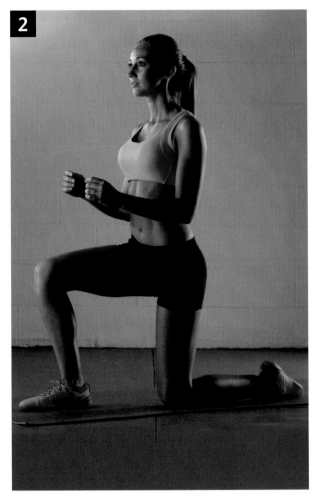

Bring your right leg forward and place your foot on the floor in front of you. Your leg should be bent at 90 degrees and your thigh should be parallel to the floor.

TRAINER TIP

The faster you can go, the higher you'll raise your heart rate. Just remember, form first and speed second.

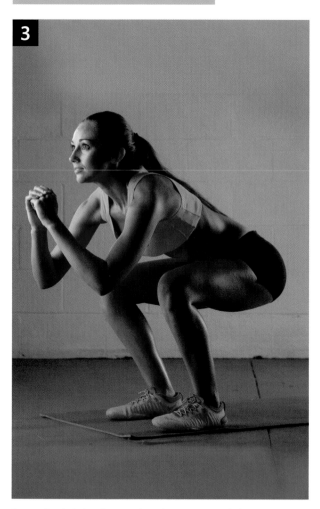

3

Bring the left leg forward and place the left foot next to the right. You should now be in a squat position with both legs bent at 90 degrees and thighs parallel to the floor.

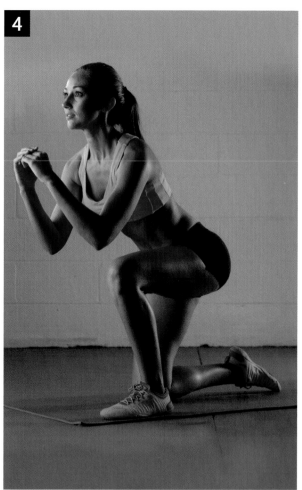

4

Return right leg to kneeling position, followed by left leg. Repeat, alternating the lead leg.

SQUAT LIFT

Develop buns of steel with this take on the traditional bodyweight squat. Adding a lateral leg lift super-charges this exercise by challenging the hips, glutes, and stabilizing leg.

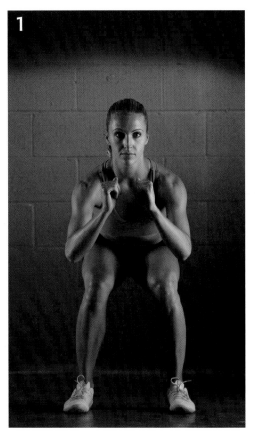

Stand tall, feet shoulder-width apart and toes pointing forward. With your weight in your heels, inhale as you bend at the knee and lower into a squat position.

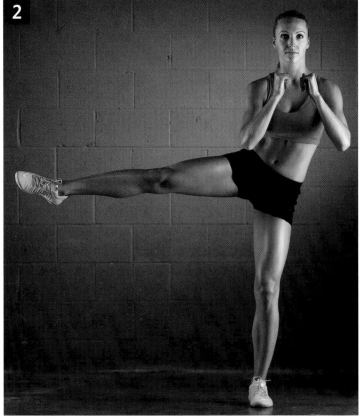

Exhale as you press through your heels. Squeeze your glutes as you stand, lifting one leg to the side as high as possible and keeping your weight on the standing leg. Keep your knees facing forward.

CHALLENGE

For an added challenge, bend the lifted leg at the knee and pull your shoulder and elbow toward the lifted leg, working your obliques.

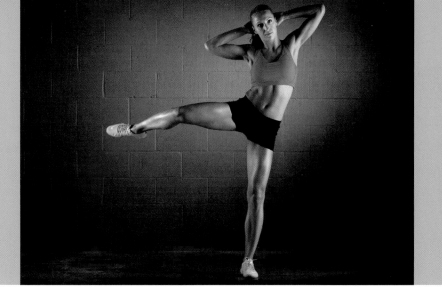

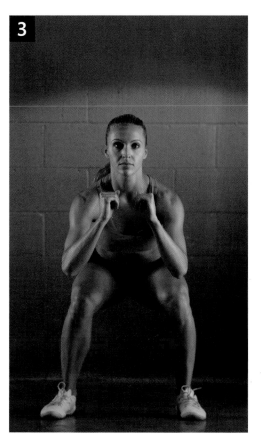

Lower your leg and return to the squat position.

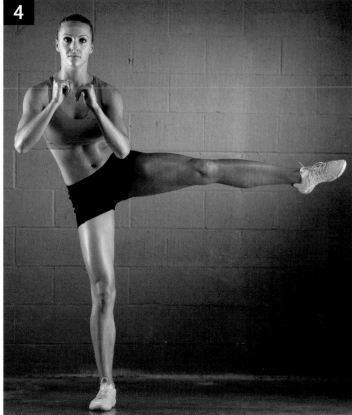

Repeat, this time lifting the opposite leg.

ROTATED DONKEY KICK

Donkey kicks work your core, lower back, and legs. With every lift you tone three butt muscles (*gluteus maximus*, *gluteus medius*, and *gluteus minimus*) giving you a firmer, rounder butt.

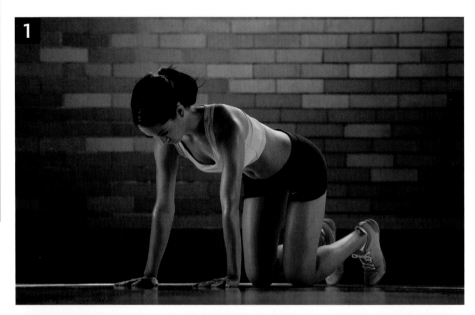

Begin on all fours with hands shoulder-width apart and knees directly below your hips. Keep your knees bent, feet flexed, and abs tight.

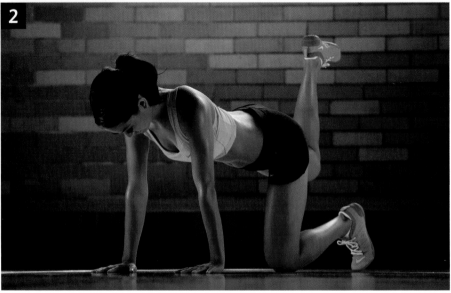

Lift one leg straight up behind you until the thigh is parallel to the floor.

TRAINER TIP

Begin slowly with discrete movements. Once you've mastered the exercise, move through the positions more quickly: lift, rotate, kick, lower.

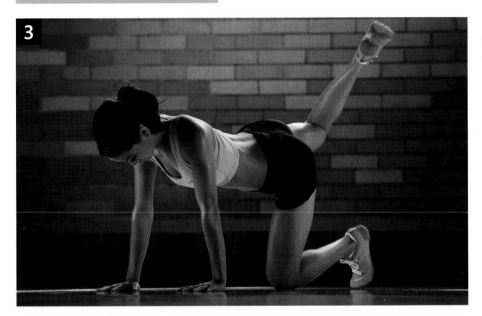

Rotate the knee so that your shin is at a 45-degree angle to the floor.

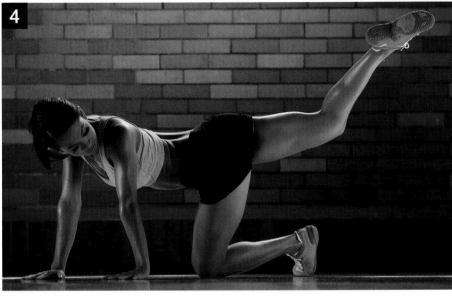

Kick your foot across the body. Look over your shoulder and imagine bringing your heel to your forehead. Return to the starting position.

LATERAL SWEEP

The lateral sweep is a ballet-inspired movement that requires core stabilization and works the obliques, hips, and thighs.

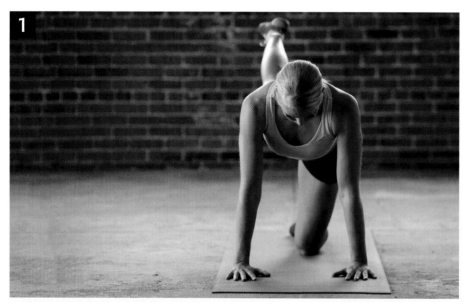

Begin on all fours, with your hands shoulder-width apart and knees directly below your hips. Extend your right leg, holding the hip high. Engage your core by pulling the belly button to the spine.

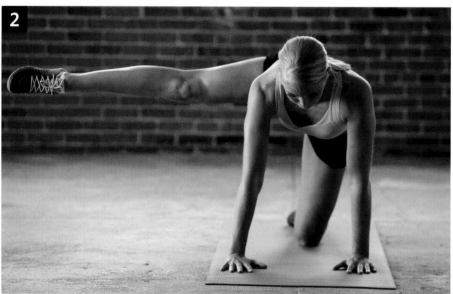

Bring the right leg forward until it is perpendicular with your body. Don't bend your elbows or arch your back.

Control the leg back to the starting position and repeat with the opposite leg.

REVERSE LUNGE

The reverse lunge is a simple, low impact way to strengthen the quads, hamstrings, glutes, and calves.

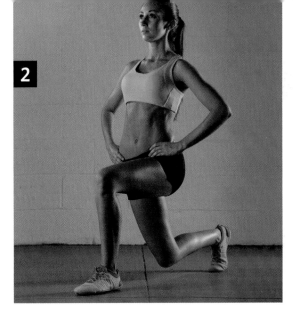

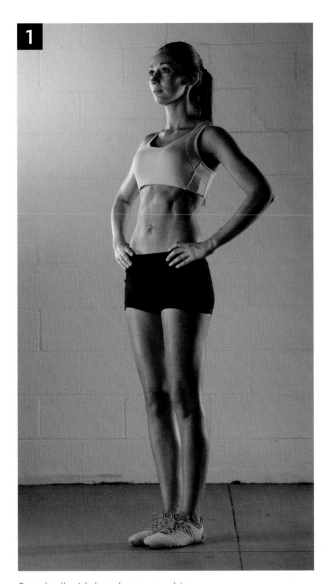

Take a large step back with your right foot. Lower your hips so that that your left thigh is parallel to the floor and your left knee is directly over your ankle. Your right knee should be bent at 90 degrees, pointing to the floor and directly under your hip.

Stand tall with hands on your hips.

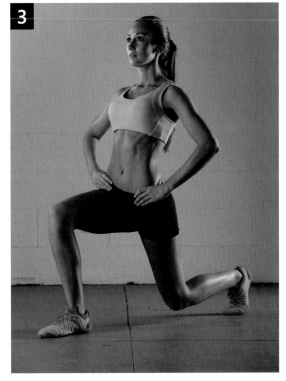

Return to a standing position and repeat, this time leading with the right leg.

INDEX

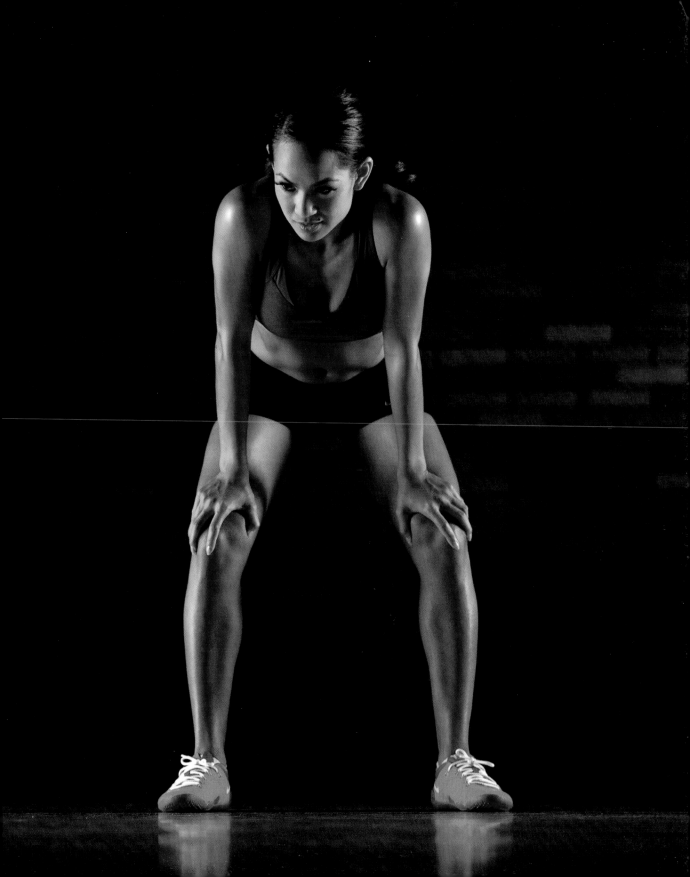

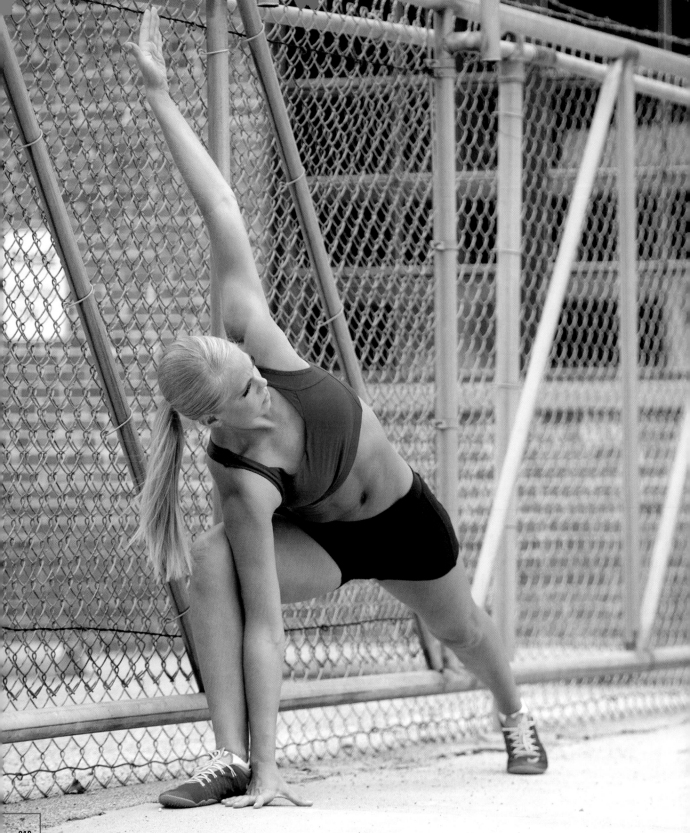

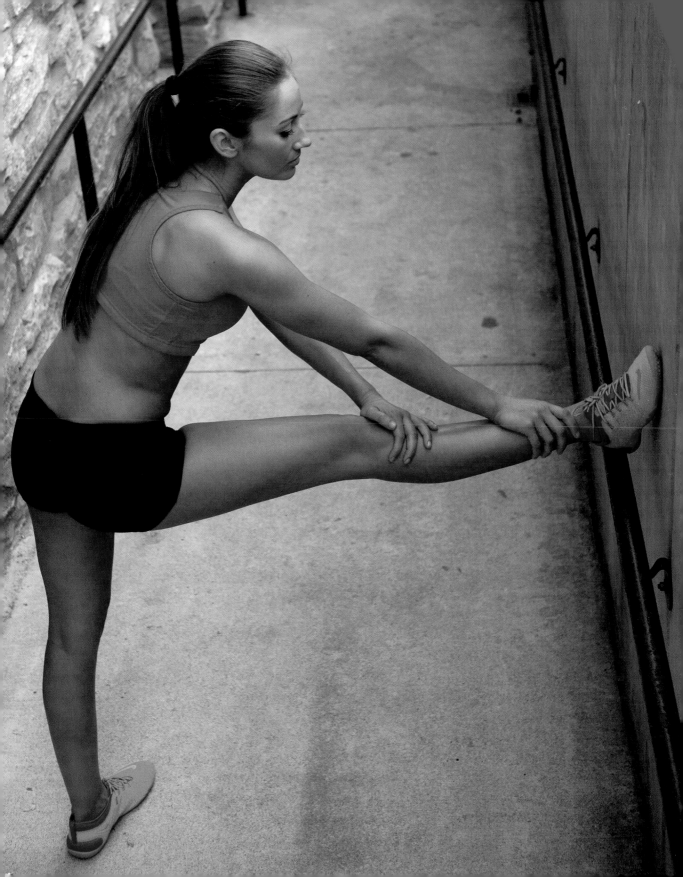

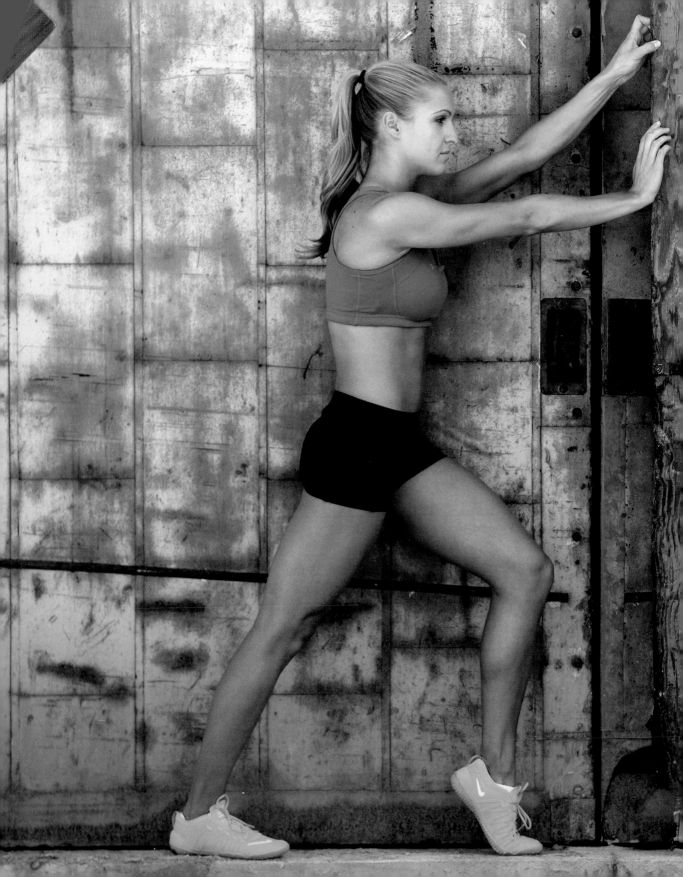